Budd
Book of Sleep

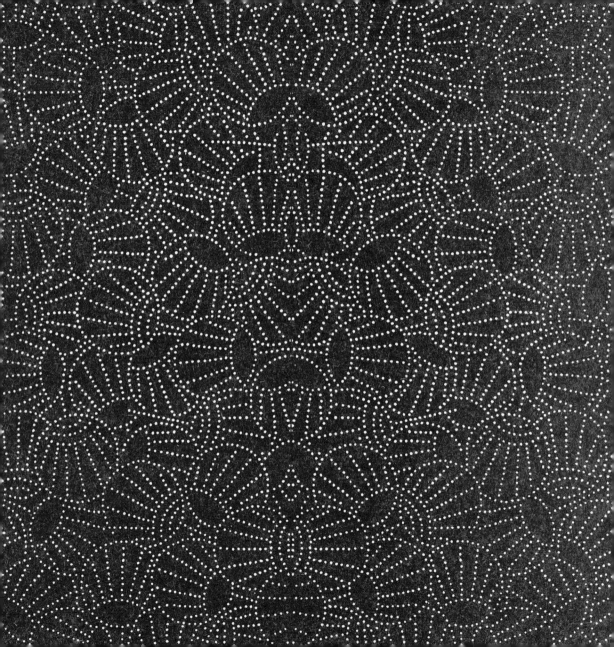

Buddha's Book of Sleep

SLEEP BETTER IN SEVEN WEEKS
with MINDFULNESS MEDITATION

Joseph Emet

JEREMY P. TARCHER
a member of Penguin Group (USA) Inc. New York

JEREMY P. TARCHER/PENGUIN
Published by the Penguin Group
Penguin Group (USA) Inc., 375 Hudson Street, New York, New York 10014, USA • Penguin Group
(Canada), 90 Eglinton Avenue East, Suite 700, Toronto, Ontario M4P 2Y3, Canada (a division of Pearson Penguin
Canada Inc.) • Penguin Books Ltd, 80 Strand, London WC2R 0RL, England • Penguin Ireland, 25 St Stephen's
Green, Dublin 2, Ireland (a division of Penguin Books Ltd) • Penguin Group (Australia), 707 Collins Street,
Melbourne, Victoria 3008, Australia (a division of Pearson Australia Group Pty Ltd) • Penguin Books India Pvt
Ltd, 11 Community Centre, Panchsheel Park, New Delhi–110 017, India • Penguin Group (NZ), 67 Apollo Drive,
Rosedale, Auckland 0632, New Zealand (a division of Pearson New Zealand Ltd) • Penguin Books, Rosebank
Office Park, 181 Jan Smuts Avenue, Parktown North 2193, South Africa • Penguin China, B7 Jaiming Center,
27 East Third Ring Road North, Chaoyang District, Beijing 100020, China

Penguin Books Ltd, Registered Offices: 80 Strand, London WC2R 0RL, England

Most Tarcher/Penguin books are available at special quantity discounts for bulk purchase for sales
promotions, premiums, fund-raising, and educational needs. Special books or book excerpts also can
be created to fit specific needs. For details, write Penguin Group (USA) Inc. Special Markets,
375 Hudson Street, New York, NY 10014.

Neither the publisher nor the author is engaged in rendering professional advice or
services to the individual reader. The ideas, procedures, and suggestions contained in this book are
not intended as a substitute for consulting with your physician. All matters regarding your health
require medical supervision. Neither the author nor the publisher shall be liable or responsible for
any loss or damage allegedly arising from any information or suggestion in this book.

ISBN 978-0-399-16091-2

Printed in the United States of America
5   7   9   10   8   6   4

BOOK DESIGN BY JESS MORPHEW

To

Thich Nhat Hanh with gratitude.

I remember:

"Happiness is not built of bricks and stones,

let us sing with the flower and the morning birds."

Children's castles; lovers' footprints
the agony of drying starfish
all gone
as the surf wipes clean the beach
with fresh waves coming from the vastness of the ocean.

Let the breath wipe away yesterday's words
this morning's thoughts
and the tightness that remains of them
until there is only this moment's freshness.

—J. E.

Contents

PART ONE
Mindfulness Meditation Training and Its Relevance for Better Sleep

PART TWO
Guided Meditation Exercises—Seven Weeks Toward Mastering Mindfulness Meditation

Foreword

I imagine that the Buddha slept peacefully, without anxiety and without worry. I think that he was peaceful in heart and mind, not only during his waking hours, but also when he lay down to sleep. The key to peaceful sleep is a peaceful mind, and the Buddha had a peaceful mind.

Knowing how to rest is an art. Without mindfulness, our propensity to be in the future instead of in the present, our habit of constantly being in our thoughts and constantly thinking about our projects, can make us exhausted. It can interfere with our ability to sleep. We can easily lose the proper balance between activity and rest.

The practice of mindfulness meditation can help to bring peace to our hearts and minds. It can alleviate stress. It can help us to slow down in order to enjoy each moment of our lives. And it can calm an agitated mind. As you read this book and do the guided meditation exercises in it, you may experience many moments of insight into the causes of your sleep difficulties. You may also learn how to relax, and improve your sleep.

—Thich Nhat Hanh

Plum Village, France

Preface

Consider the following statements:

> I know I shouldn't think about work once I'm in bed, but I do, and I get all worked up.

> I know I should not get so angry with my children, but I can't help it.

> I know I should not get second helpings at dinner, but I do, and I keep gaining weight.

> I know I should not smoke, but I continue to do it.

> I know I shouldn't let little things get to me, but I think about them when I'm in bed, and it keeps me awake.

Do any of these sound familiar? The "I" in these situations is the conscious mind. The conscious mind knows, but is unable to pass its knowledge on to the unconscious mind so that it can become second nature. Mindfulness Meditation Training (MMT) gives us the tools to pass on the knowledge of the conscious mind to the unconscious mind.

Regrets, worries, anger, and food cravings sneak up on us. With some

MMT under our belt, we can see them coming. When they knock on the door, we do not have to let them in. MMT does not make us perfect. It makes it easier to live with our imperfections. After the training, you may still feel cravings. But you are no longer a slave to your cravings. When you get into bed at night, you may still feel thoughts of all kinds trying to get into your mind. But now you have enough awareness to see them coming, and enough freedom to say, "Not now, thank you."

This may sound too good to be true. Yet countless people have been helped by mindfulness meditation training to lower their stress levels, improve their relationships, and overcome personal difficulties. This book applies similar successful techniques to achieving better sleep.

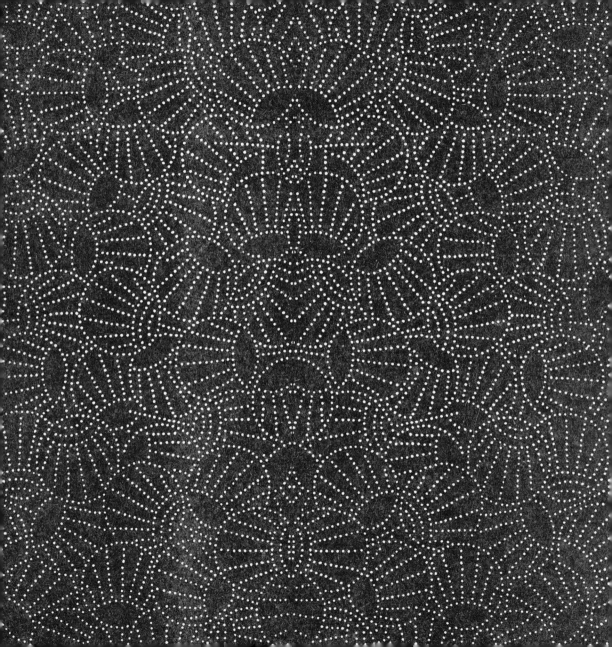

PART ONE

Mindfulness Meditation Training and Its Relevance for Better Sleep

Introduction

can hear you chuckling as you read the title of this book. You're probably thinking "Isn't Buddha better known for promoting *awakening* rather than *sleeping?*"

Yes . . . but the word *awakening* is used by Buddhists in a metaphoric sense, and used that way, it means *awareness*. For example, one may say that we seem to be asleep to the fact that we are damaging the environment with our way of life, and that we need to awaken. (In fact, we do need a rude awakening in that area.) As metaphor, *asleep* means *unconscious* or *unaware*. But the reality of sleep is different; it is a basic need like food and water, and it is the reality of sleep that this book addresses. In that sense, sleeping and awakening are not incompatible. Buddha was not promoting insomnia. On the contrary; he was promoting release from suffering, and insomnia is a form of suffering. As you do the exercises in the second part of the book, you will *awaken* to many areas of your own life while enjoying better sleep.

In one of the first mindfulness meditation groups I taught, a woman told me that she was there because she did not sleep well. She asked if mindfulness practice would help her sleep better. She was far from alone, as I discovered later. According to a 2005 survey, 75 percent of us have some kind of sleep problem. A sleep problem is not unrelated to other problems such as anxiety, worry, regret, depression, anger, and stress. These problems do not just suddenly disappear when we hit the pillow at night. They turn into sleep problems.

Sometimes it is not a Problem with a capital P that causes sleep disturbance, but a common habit we all have: the habit of mentally being somewhere else or doing something else. When discussing this issue in a group, a participant related this story: One day after work, she was driving home. She parked the car in the driveway and turned off the motor, and then realized that she was sitting in the driveway of the house she had sold six months ago.

Another participant, a teacher, told the story of having lunch in the school cafeteria one day. After lunch, the trays with the dirty dishes were to be returned to a rack. That day he found himself in the washroom face-to-face with the urinal while still holding his tray.

These stories are amusing stories of mindlessness—of doing one thing while thinking of something else. In contrast, mindfulness seeks to keep body and mind together. While thinking of something else, you can miss an exit on the highway, or worse. Nobody knows what proportion of highway accidents are caused by drivers whose minds are elsewhere. The mind has a habit of putting the body on autopilot, and then leaving to think of other things. When it starts to do that in bed, you are in trouble, because the body does not know the difference between actually having an argument, or just mentally having an argument. In both cases it gets all worked up, and the prospect of a peaceful sleep slowly evaporates.

Consider the comfort of your bed. Are you there to enjoy it? Or are you mentally somewhere else, stressing about something that happened during the day or might happen tomorrow?

Consider the mind that is always going, the mind that knows no rest. As we train that mind to get in touch with the breath and calm down, sleep becomes a possibility.

Consider our usual way of confronting the future with some anxiety. As we learn to look at tomorrow with a smile, sleep also smiles at us.

And consider our concerns about our health, relationships, children, and work. As we change our attitudes and relax our need to control everything, those concerns lose their grip on us, and we can sleep better at night. During the day, mindfulness practice can bring a sense of contentment, peace, and happiness. At night, these feelings translate into a relaxed attitude and better sleep.

I trained in mindfulness meditation with the Zen Master Thich Nhat Hanh in Plum Village, France, and was appointed a Dharma teacher by him. For the past fifteen years, I have been teaching the practice of mindfulness meditation to groups and individuals in Montreal, Canada. During this time, a few thousand people have participated in my groups. This book is a result of that experience, of the many questions I have had to answer, the many stimulating conversations I have had, and the many things the participants have forced me to consider and reconsider.

If you have some experience with mindfulness meditation, this book will show you how to apply what you already know to achieving a night of restful sleep. If you know nothing about meditation, the first part of this book will help you to transform some attitudes that you may have that are getting in the way. Our worldview has a lot to do with our ability to relax and allow sleep to take over. It is difficult to sleep on a battlefield. I would also be worried and sleepless in such a place. On a battlefield, sleeplessness is a natural response with survival value.

How do *you* see the world?

The second part of the book contains seven guided meditation exercises that nail down those attitude changes and turn them into mental habits. This part is designed as a complete course where you do each exercise for a whole week. If you want to go faster, you can try a different exercise each night of the week, and you will get an overview within the week. This makes it easy to customize the book according to your own needs. If you like one exercise more than others, for example, feel free to stick with it for a while, and move on to another exercise when you are ready. However, you will still need several weeks of practice to overcome old habits and form new ones.

Sleep is not a new skill that we have to learn. We only have to be *aware* of how we prevent ourselves from sleeping and stop whatever we are doing that gets in the way. That is why mindfulness practice, which is based on awareness, is a good remedy for sleep problems.

The following two examples from literature and song describe how profoundly what happens during the day affects our sleep.

try sleeping with a bad conscience

Methought I heard a voice cry "Sleep no more!
Macbeth does murder sleep"—the innocent sleep . . .
Chief nourisher in life's feast . . .
"Macbeth shall sleep no more!"

—*Macbeth*, Act 2, Scene 2

In Shakespeare's historical tragedy, Macbeth, who is a successful general in the Scottish army, murders Duncan, the king of Scotland, while Duncan is staying in Macbeth's castle in Inverness. Macbeth's wife, Lady Macbeth, is his accomplice: not only does she persuade him to do the deed, but she places bloody daggers on the guards in order to frame them for the murder. Duncan's murder sets in motion a chain of other murders. It also ruins Macbeth's sleep and the sleep of his wife, who is so disturbed by her guilty conscience that she eventually commits suicide.

Before her suicide, Lady Macbeth's symptoms become acute: she is sleep-walking, and compulsively rubbing imaginary blood off her hands for fifteen minutes at a time, repeating the memorable line, "Out damned spot, out!" A doctor is called to her bedside. To his credit, he confesses, "This disease is beyond my practice. . . . Unnatural deeds do breed unnatural troubles." (Act 5, Scene 1)

"try sleeping with a broken heart"

This is the title of a bittersweet song by Alicia Keys, who was named the top R & B artist of the decade by *Billboard* magazine. Here is how it begins:

> Even if you were a million miles away
> I could still feel you in my bed
> Near me, touch me, feel me

It is clear that the brokenhearted person has not yet let go mentally. She is still hanging on to her love, to old times and sweet memories. What makes this an outstanding song is the touching description of a wish to let go, alternating with moments of wanting to hang on.

As we read her words, we get the impression that this is not the best way to go to sleep with a broken heart. There are too many conflicting feelings.

Once we give the mind free rein, especially in a time of stress, we can drown in a drama of our own making. This is a good way to make oneself miserable. Sometimes the mind can be our worst enemy.

The song describes this situation well.

In both of these examples, the *mind* is the cause of the sleep disturbance. The mind is disturbed and agitated by what happened and must be calmed before sleep can come. Although most of us will not be implicated in such extraordinary circumstances as in Shakespeare's play, we all know regret, worry, and heartache. We all know an agitated mind. The recommendations found in popular sleep books, such as not to drink alcohol before bed and to control the sleeping environment, though useful in their way, do not address this issue. Mindfulness training does.

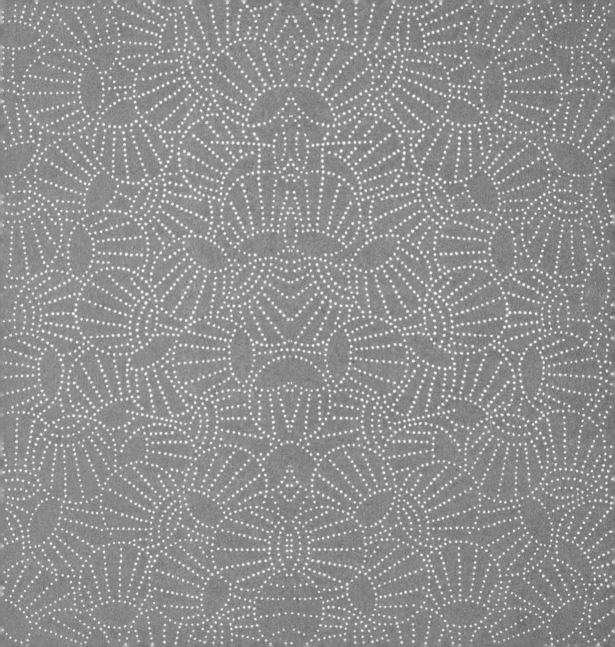

CHAPTER ONE

Mindfulness—
A New Approach

You noticed that you have a sleep problem. Perhaps you discussed it with your doctor or tried some medications, and still the problem persists. You read some books on the subject, followed the recommendations, gave up smoking, coffee, alcohol before bed, made other beneficial changes, and you are careful with your sleeping environment. And the problem is still there. You are finally face-to-face with yourself, with your mind.

This book begins where many other sleep books leave off. The problem is coming from a deeper place, and just trying to relieve the symptom is not working. Mindfulness Meditation Training is the path of awareness and self-knowledge. We come into this world without a user's manual. We have to discover the art of wise living for ourselves. In mindfulness meditation, we sit and observe what happens. If we persist, we may soon start making discoveries about our mental habits and about how our minds work. Approached this way, mindfulness practice can be an exciting path of self-discovery as new insights unfold continuously, sometimes with each meditation period.

discovery one: the busy mind

One of the first discoveries we make when we sit down to meditate is what a busy place our mind is. The heart beats, the lungs breathe, and the brain thinks. Constantly. Thinking goes on all the time. It does not stop after we hand in that brilliant term paper, finish our lesson plans for tomorrow's classes, or mail in our income taxes. Thinking does not stop when we go to bed. There is no "off" button.

Some people who start mindfulness meditation classes become overwhelmed with the sheer abundance of their own thoughts. They find it disagreeable to sit with all that confusion. Yet we cannot avoid or ignore that initial confusion. We have already found that we cannot sleep with it. Pushing it away by seeking distractions is self-limiting: the movie is soon over, the novel ends, friends leave. Eventually we need to face it and find a way to deal with it.

concentration and meditation

We start the process of MMT by concentrating on the breath.

To some this may sound simplistic. We are used to solving problems by thinking. We are not used to solving problems by breathing. Yet, if you read the first sentence again, you may now notice the word *concentrating*. We are not only breathing. In mindfulness meditation we are *concentrating* on our breath. In many traditions, concentration is synonymous with meditation. In the Thai language, *samadhi*—the word for concentration—*means* meditation.

When you really concentrate, there is nothing for you except the object of your concentration. Think tightrope walking. The rope is stretched between two tall buildings. When you really concentrate on your breath, there is nothing for you but the breath. Thoughts go out of focus. You will find that what initially sounded counterintuitive really works. If it stops working, that would be because you have lost your concentration. If you lose your balance while tightrope walking, you would not blame the rope, would you?

This concentration addresses a common situation: although your body is here, your mind may often be somewhere else. It is unconnected to your body. However, it is the body that breathes, and the mind that concentrates. Concentration on the breath brings body and mind together. As your concentration gets stronger, you may physically experience a shift in your sense of self from up in your head where the thoughts are located, to down around the chest, and finally to your belly. The expanding and contracting diaphragm is the home of the breath.

The body is our home. Thoughts are made of some kind of mental electricity; they are like an aurora borealis that comes and goes, shape-shifts, drifts, and disappears. But the body is still here through all this. As we keep our concentration on the breath, the mind is finally wrenched free from thoughts that try to take us somewhere else. We are just sitting here quietly, doing nothing, and the breath slows down and gets deeper. Before, the breath was following the random and staccato rhythm of our thoughts. Now the opposite happens: our thoughts begin to follow the steady and slow rhythm of the breath. A feeling of calm comes, and we slow down.

Concentration did not come easily to me. It may not come easily to you. Meditation periods often begin and end with a bell. When I first started meditating, the final bell would ring, and I would sometimes feel lost, as if I did not know where I was anymore. I had allowed myself to drift on wings of thought to other places. I remember many such meditation periods. Sometimes we have issues that disturb us and our concentration. At first, we may not even be aware of what those issues are. We notice only that we are not concentrating well. Mindfulness meditation gradually reveals those issues, and helps us resolve them. In turn, our concentration gets better.

I tried meditating with different groups, but the pattern was similar: meditation periods were silent and long. While this is appropriate for an advanced meditator, for many beginners it does not work well. I felt there had to be a better way to start meditation practice, and I resolved to find it. The short, guided meditation exercises in the second part of this book are the result of this search. In guided meditation, you are not left to your own devices. It is like being led through a new city by a tour guide who knows the territory. After following these exercises for some weeks, you will be ready to enjoy silent meditation periods even when they are long.

discovery two: automatic thoughts

Thinking is highly valued in our culture. I remember how surprised I was, when I first started learning about mindfulness practice, to hear thinking referred to as a burden rather than an achievement. However, this is not because mindfulness teachers are retrograde or antiachievement. There are many instances in Buddhist literature where thinking is celebrated as right thinking, clear thinking, and insight.

We usually think that we produce thoughts. It would be equally true to follow the lead of the Buddha and consider that thoughts produce us: thoughts create our sense of self, whether we view ourselves as a success or failure, for example. And many of these thoughts occur spontaneously, automatically. This was what Thich Nhat Hanh was referring to when he said, at a retreat, that only about 10 percent of our thoughts are useful.

We may be aware of that 10 percent of the purposive thought that goes into filling out an income tax form, for example, but much of our automatic thinking goes on under the radar: we may even not be aware of it happening. I would like to open a parenthesis here, and mention that one of the purposes of the concentration on the breath with which the practice of mindfulness starts is to create a general awareness of all the things we do automatically. Thich Nhat Hanh also promotes walking meditation, eating meditation, and even "dish-washing meditation." As we turn our gaze inward to observe these activities consciously, our automatic thoughts and even our emotions begin to come into focus. We start to live consciously.

Automatic thinking can cause many problems. Cognitive behavioral therapy focuses on instances where our thinking causes us grief when it is unrealistically negative or unwarranted. But the problems do not stop there. Spontaneous thinking can cause problems just by its sheer profusion. I can remember instances when thinking about something that went perfectly well and gloating over my success prevented me from sleeping! And there is more: automatic thinking also prevents us from listening to others.

Say you are listening to your spouse. Perhaps *listening* is not even the right word here. Let's just say that your spouse is talking, and you *look* as if you are listening. But, in fact, your mind is not just quietly taking in what is being said. It may be evaluating, jumping to conclusions, thinking about other things, thinking about what you are going to say when it is your turn to speak . . . it is almost as if you are thinking with the sound turned off. In some cultures, they often do not even bother to turn the sound off as they think. Often everybody just talks at the same time. There is much talking, but little listening. True listening is an art. It is achieved after we first become aware of this habit, and consciously make space so that we can hear what is being said. Otherwise, despite all the talking, communication may not be happening.

Some people become aware of how much they think only at bedtime, or when they attempt meditation for the first time. I have even encountered a few who thought that meditation *causes* this phenomenon. It is not surprising that when these people face sleep difficulties, they have the impression that the problems came out of the blue.

discovery three: negative thoughts

Often a good part of our automatic thinking is negative. Discontent comes naturally to us. Kids are discontented with their parents, parents are discontented with their teenagers, we are all discontented with our weight, and the prevalence of aesthetic surgery points to our discontent with the way we look. It is as if the brain is wired for discontent.

With mindfulness we can be aware of this tendency. I remember distinctly the first time I became aware of my habit of negative thinking. I was at a staff meeting at work. All of a sudden, I noticed that I had a negative mental comment about most people who spoke. Either he was incompetent, or he kept saying the same useless things, or he did not really understand the problem. This discovery hit me strongly at the time. Then I got caught up with work and forgot about it.

Some time later, I was at a Buddhist retreat, the distractions of the work environment were not there, and I was alone with my mind. Once again, I suddenly noticed that many things were done wrong: the schedule was wrong, we were getting up too early, the meals were poorly organized, the talks were not very good. Then a light bulb went on: Maybe the problems were in my mind rather than out there. Maybe I had difficulty accepting things as they are, and people as they are. This time there was nothing to distract me, and I was able to explore this mental habit fully and see how it was interfering with my enjoyment of the retreat.

In these last two examples, the negative thoughts were about the present, and represent one of my own mental habits as I experienced it some time ago. Other people have different mental habits. Their negative thoughts may be about the future in the form of worry or anxiety. They can also be about themselves and give rise to a lack of self-confidence or lack of self-appreciation.

negative thoughts at bedtime

During the day there are many distractions. Things are happening, there are people around, a computer on the desk, phone calls, or all of the above. But at bedtime, we are alone with our thoughts. Instead of being in small print as they were during the day negative thoughts are now written in large banners. We can no longer ignore them or take comfort in confiding to a fellow worker or a friend, as we can during the day.

Usually when people become interested in finding a way to improve their sleeping, they look at what happens after the lights go out. But if your mind has been full of negative thoughts all day, is there a way to suddenly become a positive thinker when the lights are out? Negative thoughts create their own negative emotions, such as fear and anger. These can keep us awake.

One category of negative thoughts that is particularly bothersome at bedtime is worrying *about* sleep. This is some kind of performance anxiety, like worrying about sexual performance, or even like worrying about a musical performance onstage, the so-called *stage fright*. And it is just as counterproductive. Worrying about whether you will be able to sleep, or whether you will be able to sleep well, or sleep enough, creates the same negative consequences as other kinds of worrying, plus it makes some people try to control sleep. This backfires. I still own a lapel button that made the rounds in the eighties. It asks, "Are we having fun yet?" Constantly asking yourself, "Have I started to fall asleep yet?" when you are in bed can be a little bit like wearing that button to a party! The issue of control is more thoroughly discussed in chapter 3.

One antidote to negative emotions is gratitude.

gratitude heals

I am grateful for what I am and have. My thanksgiving is perpetual.

It is surprising how contented one can be with nothing definite—only a sense of existence.

My breath is sweet to me. O how I laugh when I think of my vague, indefinite riches.

My wealth is not possession but enjoyment.

—HENRY DAVID THOREAU

Gratitude is the opposite of dissatisfaction. Gratitude is the ability to find what is right among things that may be going wrong, and to appreciate it. Every day something must be going right, because we are still alive. Life is a miracle of sorts. Science does not quite understand it. Gratitude for this miracle is an appropriate response.

Contentment and gratitude are wonderful things to focus on at bedtime. Your mind needs something to chew on. Instead of letting it chew on any old bone that turns up on the scrap heap, give it a juicy morsel: count your blessings. It is more satisfying than counting sheep or watching the evening news. You may have heard the saying, "No news is good news." Most of the time the networks follow the philosophy that the only news worth reporting is bad news. Not only is this inappropriate bedtime material, it is actually skewed reporting. At bedtime, we need to hear what is right with the world. A generation or two ago, many people ended the day with an evening prayer rather than with the evening news. The good feelings generated by prayer made it easier to let go and relax into sleep. The evening news often has the opposite effect.

A gratitude exercise begins with taking stock of all the good things in our life and appreciating them. However, the first time you try it, nothing may occur to you right away. This is okay. You may need to dig deeper, and you may need practice. Thinking of negatives may have become a habit.

For example, you think of your spouse, and the first thing that jumps into your mind is something he does that irritates you. (Please switch genders as the situation demands.) Just put that aside for a moment, and make a b-i-g effort to think of something he did that you enjoyed. If nothing comes to mind, just stay with the question until something does come to you. It could be a small thing. Nothing is too small for this exercise. Once you start, even with a small item, other positive things will follow. Soon, you will be surprised at what a great guy he is. Go ahead, and allow yourself to feel thankful for having him as a partner. This exercise will help put that one irritating item in perspective. In the end, you will find that it is much easier to sleep knowing that you are living with someone you appreciate. You can do that systematically with your children, your neighbors, or your boss. After a few weeks of gratitude practice, you may be surprised that when you think of someone now, it is the good things that jump to your mind first instead of the negatives. You think of people with a smile. And what you did to sleep better at night may end up improving your relationships during the day, because when you look at someone with appreciation and love in your eyes, they tend to reciprocate.

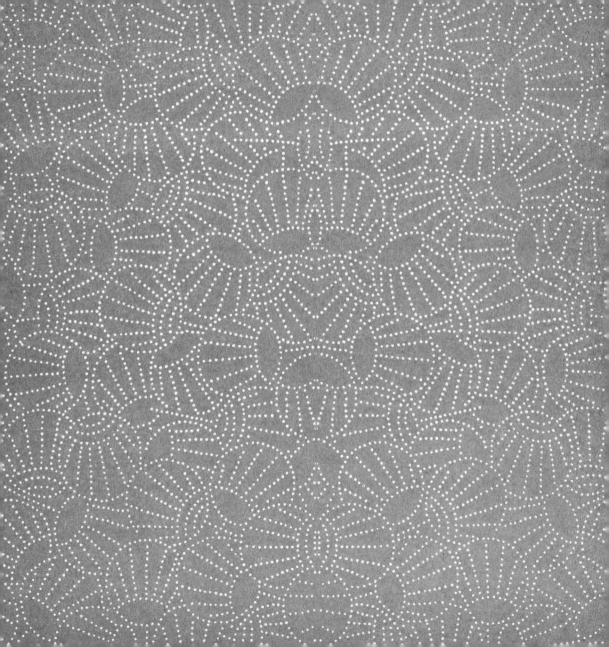

CHAPTER TWO

During the Night

the twilight zone

With this chapter, we move to what happens between bedtime and wake-up time, specifically to waking up before wake-up time.

Often there is a twilight zone between sleep and wakefulness—we are asleep, but we are thinking almost as if we are awake. We may be thinking thoughts like, "I should get up and close the window," or, "I should get up and go to the bathroom." Another common one is "I should get up and ask them to turn down the noise." In the twilight zone, we can either wake ourselves up or continue sleeping.

Something similar sometimes happens during meditation. If you are meditating alone at home, you might get an urge to go raid the fridge, or to pick up the phone when it rings. My favorite is the urge to scratch my nose.

As I write these lines, I'm reminded of the time when my partner was the owner of a bakery. One night around 1:00 a.m., the phone rang. It was the police. The bakery had been broken into, the plate glass was smashed, and the cash register was lying on the floor with the drawer open. She held the phone to her ear for a moment, and softly mumbled something like, "Thank you, I will deal with it in the morning." She then turned the other way and was asleep again. I was awestruck by her ability to do that. She did not allow the police officer's story to disturb her. As she later explained to me, "What else is left to steal, muffins?"

Knowing the difference between a disturbance, such as pain or noise, on the one hand, and our feelings around these, on the other hand, is another aspect of mindfulness practice. The person who continues to sleep through a disturbance might be aware of the sounds at some level, but does not get worked up about them. She might know that the snowplow passed and the garbage truck went by, even though she continues to sleep.

How does meditation practice help us sleep through a disturbance?

Disturbances also occur during sitting meditation. These run the gamut from an itchy nose, to discomfort in the legs, to write an e-mail. Painful feelings may also come up. In meditation we learn to sit with whatever comes up. Meditation puts a little buffer zone between thoughts and actions. Instead of immediately gratifying such urges, we learn to acknowledge them, smile at them, and continue sitting. This habit is invaluable when we are angry: that little buffer zone is quite precious when we get an urge to act in a certain way out of anger. It is also helpful during the twilight zone: we do not take every thought that passes through our mind as a clue to bound out of bed and do something. Our attitude during meditation may go something like this:

Breathing in and out, I'm aware of a certain discomfort in my legs.
I smile at the discomfort and continue to enjoy my breathing.

Substitute "craving for ice cream" for "certain discomfort in the legs," and the practice becomes:

Breathing in and out, I'm aware of a craving for ice cream.
I smile at my craving and continue to enjoy my breathing.

You can see the relevance of this practice for weight control.

Substitute "a certain noise," and the practice now becomes:

Breathing in and out, I'm aware of a certain noise.
I smile at the noise and continue to enjoy my breathing.

You can also substitute "irritation" if that is a bigger issue for you:

Breathing in and out, I'm aware of a certain irritation.
I smile at the irritation and continue to enjoy my breathing.

Now you can see the relevance of this kind of practice for the twilight zone. As we learn to hold a certain discomfort, craving, or irritation without reacting, we gain freedom. External events do not control us as much anymore, and we do not act in a knee-jerk sort of way. This has benefits in many areas of our lives.

waking up in the dark

If you have a tendency to wake up at, say, three in the morning, first be reassured that you are not alone. Many people who are past the first bloom of youth have this tendency. A. Roger Ekirch documents in his book *At Day's*

Close that before the industrial revolution, people typically slept in two discrete phases, bridged by an intervening period of wakefulness of up to an hour or more. Peasant couples, who were often too tired after field labor to do much more than eat and go to sleep, awakened later to have sex. People also used this time to pray, reflect, or interpret dreams. This was also a favorite time for scholars and poets to write.

Ekirch's historical account was preceded by a few years by a groundbreaking study by psychiatrist Thomas Wehr. Wehr is one of the people who identified SAD (seasonal affective disorder), and he developed light therapy to treat it. In the study in question, Wehr put a group of healthy volunteers in complete darkness for fourteen hours a day for a month, and found that by the end of the month, his subjects had settled into a pattern where they slept for three to five hours, then awakened for an hour or two before a second three-to-five-hour sleep period. Perhaps so many grocery stores in the United States are open twenty-four hours a day because many of us have this tendency for polyphasic sleep.

I first became aware of how widespread polyphasic sleep is during a business trip with a friend. I had planned to pick her up early in the morning, and I was in front of her apartment building at 4:00 a.m. She lives in a high-rise that wraps around a parking lot. I rang the bell and waited. Soon, I noticed that there were flashes like lightning in the air. I looked up; the sky was clear, and I could see the stars. I looked behind, and saw that the TV was on in many of the apartments. Indeed, according to market research, plenty of viewers watch Fox News at 3:00 a.m.

When I mentioned this at a "sleep better" course I was teaching, many eyes lit up with relief. One participant, a busy executive, told me that for many years he was president of a nonprofit corporation as a volunteer, and did all the extra work this entailed when he woke up at 3:00 a.m.

Early morning is a privileged time. Spiritual traditions across many cultures know this well. Thai Forest monasteries, Zen centers, and Catholic monasteries have early wake-up schedules. At home, what we do with our time when we wake up in the middle of the night is up to us. The wide-awake period typically lasts for an hour or ninety minutes. We can watch TV or meditate. We can fuss and fume or do something useful that needs doing anyway. This is also a very good time for doing the exercises in the second part of this book.

Of course, the problem with waking up at that time is how to manage to get enough sleep. One solution is to go to bed early. But many of us don't want to do that. As children, we looked up to parents who put us to bed early and then went off to do "cool" things like watch TV. Ever since, we think that going to bed early is uncool. I occasionally see my partner groggy with sleep at 9:30 in the evening as she drags herself around for another hour, because "it is too early to go to bed yet." Going to sleep early may or may not work for you. Experiment and see.

In many Latin countries, the afternoon siesta is the norm. This charming custom must be there for a reason. So far as I can tell, the recent wave of concern about sleep deprivation comes from siesta-hostile rather than siesta-friendly countries. If you are predisposed to take siestas, you may find yourself like a square peg in a round hole in the nine-to-five world of work.

sleep deprived or nap deprived?

If you feel sleepy in the afternoon, it may be that you need a short nap in the afternoon rather than more sleep at night. Personally, I need a twenty-minute nap to be at my best in the afternoon. An extra hour of sleep at night will not do it for me. On the other hand, my partner, Suzanne, has afternoon insomnia. She never takes a nap. She does not seem to need it. If you are like me, you may enjoy reading William A. Anthony's comments on the subject in his 1997 book, *The Art of Napping*:

> Many people do not know about the benefits of napping—another example of forgetting what we learned as children! Still other people feel guilty about their napping. They hide the fact that they do nap.

We live in a nappist society—where napping is discriminated against. Napping occurs across the age span and around the world. Most mammals nap. Lack of napping behavior is the exception, not the rule. Indeed, a majority of people nap—but they don't talk about it in public.

Dr. Anthony reports that there is no evidence that daytime napping reduces your ability to sleep at night.

perfect nights?

Here is one of my favorite Mullah Nasruddin stories. A friend once asked him why he had never married. He replied that it was because he had been looking for the perfect woman. His friend asked him what happened. The mullah recounted the story of his loves, how he had come close to marrying a few times, but found that the woman in question had some defect, such as not being kind enough, or industrious enough, or charming enough. Then he started waxing lyrical about one beauty who had all the right qualities. His friend asked the obvious question:

"So why did you not marry her?"

The mournful answer came: "Alas, she was looking for the perfect man."

What I get from this story is that if a "perfect" thing happens, enjoy it. But if you go *looking* for that perfect thing, you might never find it. Perfect things have a way of showing up on their own when they do show up. Our nights will be different from one another, just as our days are. Wanting them all to conform to a preconceived mold may only serve to create stress.

inspired nights

According to biographers of Paul McCartney and the Beatles, the entire melody of his hit song "Yesterday" came to McCartney in a dream one night while he was staying in the home of his then-girlfriend, Jane Asher. Upon waking, he went right away to a piano and played the tune to avoid forgetting it.

More recently, Lady Gaga told a television interviewer that "Sometimes in the middle of night when I'm falling asleep I have a lot of ideas, then wake up and record them into my phone and send it to my producers." Important scientific discoveries have also been made as a result of dreams. Inspiration often comes uninvited and unexpected. In the quiet of the night, we can find the space to explore the full meaning of a dream or an insight.

CHAPTER THREE

Here and Now in Bed

Weary with toil, I haste me to my bed

The dear repose for limbs with travel tired;

But then begins a journey in my head

To work my mind, when body's work's expir'd:

For then my thoughts—from far where I abide—

Intend a zealous pilgrimage to thee,

And keep my drooping eyelids open wide . . .

—WILLIAM SHAKESPEARE, FROM SONNET 27

The mindfulness mantra "Be here now" is as appropriate as a practice theme at night as it is during daytime. It is our thoughts that keep us awake. When we are in the past or in the future, we are in our thoughts. When we are here now, we are in our senses. The mind is constantly taking over from the five senses. That's how we end up being mentally somewhere else. The mind is like the bully in the playground: evolution gave us this bully. Our large and powerful brain has many advantages, but it also has a downside. The bully body checks the five senses, it takes over, and before we know it, we are in the past regretting something, or reliving some experience that happened five years ago. We might also be in the future imagining things, worrying about what might happen, or daydreaming about a pleasant possibility.

During the day, the five senses at least have a chance: the world reaches out and claims our attention. If we slip back into our thoughts while crossing the street, a car horn might jerk us back into our senses so that we do not get run over. Or a flashing red light ahead may bring us back from our thoughts to our driving. Between such moments, we still slide back into our thoughts. But it is at night that the bully is in his element. At night, he has no challengers. All is dark and quiet. Nothing to rescue us from his grip, nothing to grab our attention and bring us to the here and now. At night, the mind can exaggerate a health problem, for example, or some incident at work. Then the imagination can take over and weave a worst-case scenario that keeps us awake.

go to sleep with your eyes open

You can sometimes prevent that from happening by keeping your eyes open when you go to bed, instead of closing them in anticipation of sleep. Let sleep close your eyes, rather than your anticipation. This simple trick can sometimes make a difference, and it works even when there is just the slightest hint of light in the room, and you see only some shadows. Remember those times when you were driving or at a lecture, and you began to feel sleepy? Your eyes were open. You may even have struggled to keep them open as you felt sleepier and sleepier, and your eyelids felt heavier and heavier.

When we read in bed, that is what we are doing—we are keeping our eyes open until we begin to feel really sleepy. Babies stare at the mobile on their crib until their eyes glaze. Then, when sleep comes, the eyes just close on their own. Keeping our eyes open helps keep us in the here and now, and in our senses. That makes sleep easier. Closing the eyes in anticipation of sleep often has the opposite effect: it switches the focus of the mind from our senses to our thoughts.

confidence, not control

Our conscious mind would like to control everything: the weather, the stock market, our children, and our spouse. Yet, it cannot even control its own body. Consider the facts: You may not want to get pregnant, but you do. On the other hand, someday you may want to get pregnant, but you find that you can't. Now you are in bed and want to sleep, but you can't. Then when you are driving or listening to a lecture, you want to stay awake, but you get sleepy. You don't ever want to get sick, but you do.

Some people react to this lack of control with anxiety and worry. If they are driving, they are keenly aware that they do not control other drivers. They do not have confidence that other drivers will be careful and conscientious like them. If they are walking or crossing the street, they worry that other drivers will not stop for them. They are terrified of what may happen to their children in this out-of-control world.

At night, they feel as if they are sleeping in a lion's den.

If you are one of these people, consider that it may be a good thing that other drivers are not like you, and that when you get sleepy, they do not also get sleepy at the same time. Remember those times when other drivers have taken care of you as you made an awkward maneuver.

Consider that you are alive now due to the care and attention of others. Not only in such obvious situations as when you have been on the operating table in a hospital, but in everyday, mundane circumstances as well. Pilots and air traffic controllers have done their jobs conscientiously and have not crashed any planes that you were on. Bus and taxi drivers have driven you around with care.

The short meditation theme on page 49 is an excellent antidote for worry and fear.

But if worrying is a deeply entrenched habit for you, then the voice of the worrisome thoughts in your mind may drown out that meditation theme. That does not mean that mindfulness practice is not working. It means that you need the full regimen of MMT; you need the full seven-week practice period.

brain spam

Mindfulness practice does not make worrisome thoughts and feelings suddenly disappear. Instead, you learn to put some distance between you and your thoughts. You stop identifying with them. You do not have to take a thought to be true just because it crosses your mind. You don't have to consider each thought to be an important message. Sometimes thoughts are just spam.

We have learned to deal with spam on our computers. We have learned to ignore messages even when they are in red, flashing, or dancing about to attract our attention. But we often react to the messages coming from our own brain without considering the possibility that they could be spam. Brain spam can be just as abundant and persuasive sounding as computer spam. With mindfulness, we can develop the habit of just letting it be without letting it disrupt our peace of mind.

Consider what makes computer spam compelling: it appeals to our greed, or to our fears. I still remember the first message I got telling me of the millions of dollars I had just received from a distant relative. Greed made me read it. I also remember the first time I got a message about a close friend who lost all his documents to theft while traveling in London, and urgently needed money. That was fear for his safety that made me waste time mulling over it.

If you have a tendency to worry, the spammer in your brain will exploit that weakness, and bombard you with worrisome thoughts. When that happens, take a deep breath, smile, and move on.

trying to control sleep

We do not control sleep. We can control only our mental and physical readiness for sleep. The paradox is that, with a goal such as sleep, it is better to forget about the goal, and just get into enjoying the relaxation of being in bed, and the luxury of feeling the bedsheets around our body. We can totally relish the freedom of having no obligations and nothing to do for the next several hours. We can be open to sleep, and give up all striving. That is what we *can* do. Any kind of effort or trying to force sleep can be counterproductive. It can keep us awake.

We have absorbed messages from our culture such as, "If at first you do not succeed, try harder." Such messages are valuable in certain areas—those where we are in control. For example, if we try harder, we *can* run faster. But in areas where we do not have conscious control, trying harder does not work; not only that, but it is often counterproductive. Instead of helping, the extra effort gets in the way. Sleep is one of those areas.

If sleep does not come easily or quickly, the voice of our social conditioning may badger us with thoughts like, "You are not trying hard enough." Working harder has been effective in many areas of our life. It may have helped us get through a course of study or get a promotion at work. As a result, we believe in success through hard work. We do not believe in success through giving up!

Yet, counterintuitive as it may sound, this is exactly what is needed where sleep is concerned: You can bring the proverbial horse to water, but you cannot make him drink. The conscious mind can bring us to the bed and make us lie down, but it cannot make us go to sleep. It has to learn to get out of the way and let nature take its course.

The attraction of sleeping pills is that they give us the illusion that we can control sleep. Gregg Jacobs effectively dispels this illusion in his book *Say Good Night to Insomnia*. He states, "Regular use of sleeping pills is no longer considered safe or appropriate due to their undesirable and potentially dangerous side effects." However, it is not only the side effects that make sleeping pills undesirable. Dr. Jacobs cites many studies that show that sleeping pills are not as effective as their manufacturers claim, and that they lose what effectiveness they have as we become habituated to them. More important, they do not help one to function better the next day. According to an Associated Press report, the Food and Drug Administration has sent letters to manufacturers of thirteen popular sleeping pills, requesting them to send letters to health-care providers to inform them about potential adverse events, which include sleep-driving, making phone calls, and preparing and eating food while in one's sleep.

becoming aware of emotions

We may be aware of our thoughts, but sometimes we are unaware of the underlying emotions that prompted them. Thoughts are articulate. They are like the handle of a cup. They are the part of a mental state that we can grasp, whereas emotions themselves can be slippery, and worse, often invisible. Sadness comes over us like fog "on cat's feet." Thoughts associated with sadness, however, may hit us with the force of a gale. When we are angry with someone, say, our partner or teenage son, we think and say all kinds of things—we diagnose all their real and imagined weaknesses, we think of all the bad things they ever did or said, while we may be unaware of what is obvious to any observer: our own anger.

Thoughts engage in a ping-pong game with emotions: emotions give rise to thoughts, and thoughts fuel emotions. We may be angry at someone and think, "How could she do this to me?" That thought makes us angrier, and the emotion stimulates another thought: "She is so mean." This thought in turn adds more fuel to our anger. Through all this, we may be aware only of our thoughts, but not the underlying emotion that stirs them.

This ping-pong effect is what keeps worry going. A feeling of worry or lack of confidence, by itself, will come and go "like a cloud in a windy sky," without leaving a trace. No problem. But without awareness, it gives rise to thoughts, worst-case scenarios, and conjectures of all kinds. These thoughts fuel more worry and keep us awake. Without mindfulness, we can keep nourishing our anxiety, and keep the worry orgy going all night.

We can intervene in this vicious circle. We recognize the feeling, and smile at it. We mentally say, "Hello, worry, I know that you are there." We do not nourish the feeling with thoughts. It is as if in a game, our partner threw us the ping-pong ball. Instead of hitting it back, we now grab the ball in our hand and put it in the garbage can. Game over.

Adding fuel to a fire is an appropriate metaphor for the relationship between thoughts and emotions. If we do not add fuel to a fire, it will go out. A campfire will stop burning if we stop feeding it logs and branches. Angry thoughts keep the fire of anger burning.

If You Find It Difficult to Stop Angry Thoughts, Here Are a Few Suggestions:

1. Concentrate on the breath to take your mind off your thoughts. In the second part of this book, the first exercise, Calming the Mind, will take you through the steps. If you do this exercise as recommended, you may find that the anger has subsided and the mind is calmer.
2. Use the opposite emotion to drive out anger. The opposite of anger is loving kindness. Just one drop of compassion can be enough to bring back spring in our hearts.
3. Are you angry with your teenage son? Research suggests that the teenage brain is not fully developed. Your son has an incomplete brain. It is harder to be angry with a disabled person. Thinking of him as disabled may be the drop of compassion you need to derail your anger.

Indeed, in Buddhist imagery, Avalokiteshvara, the Buddha of compassion (Quan Yin in Chinese), is pictured holding a flask of water. She has a willow branch in the other hand. She dips the willow branch into the flask and sprinkles the water of compassion on the earth. She does not have a fire hose in her hand. She does not need one. Just a few delicate drops of the metaphorical water of compassion will put out the fires of anger or hatred. If you like this metaphor and find it helpful, you can get a small statue of Quan Yin in any Chinese gift shop. Ask for "the female Buddha." Putting this statue in a prominent place in your house will remind you of the power of compassion when you need a reminder.

the worry habit

Worry can arise spontaneously in the mind. But if we dwell on it, cultivate it, and rehearse it night after night, it slowly turns into a habit. Like a weed that is lovingly watered and nourished, it grows stronger, spreads, and takes over the garden of our mind. We get better at playing worry ping-pong. Each time we allow ourselves to wallow in it instead of letting go of it as described above, worrying becomes more habitual and harder to stop.

Mindfulness practice begins with awareness of spontaneous and automatic activities such as breathing and walking. With practice, we become aware of emotions that also arise spontaneously. We become aware of them at an earlier stage. This awareness gives us choices. We do not *suddenly* find ourselves in the middle of a ping-pong game that we are powerless to stop. We do not continue to nourish the *feeling* of worry with unwarranted *thoughts* of worry.

If you do the exercises systematically as recommended, you will find this easier to do.

building trust

Consider that each day we are alive because of someone else's care and attention. Each time we cross the street, someone else is watching for us. Each time we make a left turn, someone else is careful to wait for us.

A good exercise to do at night is to make a mental list of how many times that day your life depended on others, on their care and attention. As you picture each such situation, send a mental note of thank-you and appreciation to those concerned.

After this, you can go on to situations where your life was not on the line, but other people's care and kindness made things more pleasant for you. You can send a note of appreciation to the grocery store clerks who keep the shelves stocked with fresh produce. To the city workers who keep your water running. To the power company workers who make sure that you have power.

The whole universe is cooperating in keeping us alive and well.

Babies and young children sleep easier in the presence of their parents. It is easier to let go and fall asleep in the arms of people who take care of you and in whom you have trust. We outgrow our need for parents, but we do not outgrow our need for trust.

embracing our lack of confidence with a smile

The way of mindfulness is to acknowledge a feeling and just hold it. As we do that, we may get insights into where it comes from, but for the moment we just accept it. We also accept that there is more to us than this particular feeling or emotion. We need not let it rule our life or dominate our mind. What does a lack of confidence feel like in our body and mind?

Breathing in, breathing out. I feel a lack of confidence.
I smile at my lack of confidence and continue to enjoy my breath.

The important thing is our attitude toward our feelings and emotions. They come and go. And they do not necessarily reflect reality. Confidence and the lack of it both create their own momentum. They can be self-fulfilling prophecies.

As you practice with the short meditation theme above, you may find the butterflies quieting down. If the butterflies persist, try again tomorrow, and do the exercises at the end of the book. When we were learning to walk, we fell many times. But we got up and tried again. If we had given up after the first fall, we might still be crawling today.

"i've done my best"

Is a good meditation theme at bedtime. It is an affirmation that brings contentment. Indeed, doing our best is a realistic target to aim for. It takes us conveniently out of the business of trying to control the universe.

Consider that the fruits of our actions do not depend entirely on us. They depend on many other factors—and we don't even know what they all are. A doctor could make his best effort to save the life of a patient, but the patient could still die "from unknown causes." Neither the doctor nor anyone else controls all these causes. The only thing the doctor controls is his own actions. Doing our best is all anyone can do.

trust yourself, trust others

Shunryu Suzuki's well-known book *Zen Mind, Beginner's Mind* is a collection of transcriptions of improvised talks. So is Thich Nhat Hanh's *The Path of Emancipation*. These masters of meditation were confident that, once they started to talk, the right words would come to them. Trust in the flow of inspiration makes for an exciting talk, an outstanding performance, or an inspired conversation during the day. At night, it translates into a feeling of confidence that things will be all right tomorrow and that with mindfulness most situations can be handled gracefully. We can let go with a smile, and "go gentle into that good night."

dylan thomas

Do not go gentle into that good night . . .
Rage, rage against the dying of the light.

As I recalled those repeating lines from his well-known poem, I had a hunch that the Welsh poet Dylan Thomas probably had an issue with sleep. There is a reluctance to let go in those lines, and a lack of appreciation for peace.

My hunch turned out to be correct. The poem is ostensibly about death, but the metaphor also throws light on his tortured relationship with sleep. The difficulties and problems of his waking life did not go away when Dylan Thomas went to bed. It turned to insomnia. Insomnia haunted him all his life. His biographer Paul Ferris reports that, as a boy, Thomas wrote a poem about a tormented adolescent who cannot sleep. As a young man, he slept badly and lay awake for hours. Later in life, he carried around a bottle of sleeping pills, and wrote to Caitlin, his wife, "I do not sleep until dawn." Near the end of his life, he complained that he was too tired to sleep. Sleep deprivation may have contributed to his total collapse and death at the age of thirty-nine.

CHAPTER FOUR

Suffering Is Not Enough

As Thich Nhat Hanh writes in *The Heart of the Buddha's Teaching*, for forty-five years the Buddha said, "I teach suffering and the transformation of suffering." The second part of this sentence, the part about transforming suffering, is the key to understanding the Buddha's smile. It is the smile of a man who has found the way out of suffering instead of getting stuck in it.

This core teaching of the Buddha is known as the Four Noble Truths. It is a process that starts with looking at our suffering dispassionately for once, without getting caught up in it, and seeing how we contribute to creating it.

But suffering is not enough. The next step is to stop making ourselves suffer, to let go of those attitudes and mental habits that create stress or make us unhappy. The fourth step is traditionally known as the Noble Eightfold Path. The Buddhist teacher Bhante Henepola Gunaratana refers to it as *Eight Mindful Steps to Happiness* in the title of his book on the subject. Thich Nhat Hanh sometimes calls it "the path of well-being," as it is a list of ways of living and thinking that lead to happiness. Appropriately, these include concentration and mindfulness. Concentration is an ally of mindfulness. It gives us the ability to stay with and look deeply into the knots inside so we can start the work of undoing them.

Suffering arises over and over again, either because our memories of a traumatic moment keep coming back, or simply because life never stops throwing curves at us. Separation, sickness, and aging are part of life, and they are stressful. You can practice the Four Noble Truths with each breath as you feel tension, stress, and worry.

During one of his Dharma talks, Thich Nhat Hanh remarked that His Holiness the Dalai Lama had written a book titled *The Art of Happiness*. With a smile, he then added that one day he would like to write a book called *The Art of Suffering*. What I take away from this comment is that we can either get stuck in suffering, or we can learn from suffering: we can learn to go beyond it. Artful suffering would be this ability to move beyond suffering toward happiness. Indeed, understood in this way, the art of suffering is not that different from the art of happiness. The Four Noble Truths are interdependent.

There is deep wisdom in the mindfulness motto "Be here now." If a traumatic event from the past is bothering you and keeping you awake, being here now means looking at that issue with your feet firmly planted in the present moment, from the perspective of the person you are now. When you go to the past, you get plunged back into the feelings of the past. Stay in the present moment. Bring that issue that bothers you to the present. Look at it with all the understanding and love you now have: understanding for all the people involved, and love for yourself. Transporting yourself to the past in some kind of a mental time machine takes you to the whole situation with its painful feelings. You suffer over and over again, even though that situation no longer exists. You are in a hell of your imagination. Stay here: if you have suffered as a little child, do not become that little child and suffer again. Look at the situation with the eyes you have now and heal yourself.

right diligence

This item in the Noble Eightfold Path is particularly useful in changing those habits of mind that do not bring us happiness. This item is actually a whole program with four aspects. Traditionally, these are discussed starting with the negatives. Here, I will start with positives and present them in a slightly modified way:

1. If you do not now have a positive thought in your mind, *find* something positive to think about. Gratitude is a good way to get started. Or if you are thinking of a person, you can imagine that somebody gave you an assignment to find five good things about that person. If you are thinking of your day, just make a list of all the good things that happened. Feelings and states of mind usually follow thoughts.

2. If you already have some positive thoughts or feelings, hang on to them as long as you can. For example, if you were already thinking positive thoughts about a member of your family, continue doing so. Keep on thinking positive thoughts.

3. If a negative thought shows up, acknowledge it. Then just say to your mind, "Not now, thank you," and continue with the positives.

4. If you find that the negative thought or attitude has already taken hold, accept its presence. You could take this opportunity to look deeply to find out what triggered the negative attitude and where it came from. Understanding brings peace and healing. Negative thoughts are just thoughts. They are the way we

conceptualize a situation or a person. It is possible to change them by looking at things with a more compassionate eye. When we do that, the new, more compassionate attitude drives out the old one.

This is a little bit like changing the station when we listen to the radio: When there is good music on the radio we keep listening. But if there is something that does not nourish the spirit, we can change the station. Minds are like radio stations in this regard; they can keep repeating things that do not contribute to our well-being or blabber away without saying anything worth hearing. Something better is just a breath away. For example, we may be lying in bed reflecting on the things that happened during the day. Suddenly, we may notice that we are thinking of the day's events with a "half-empty glass" attitude. By staying in a negative mental state and identifying with the thoughts it generates, we make ourselves unhappy in the present, and we also boost the ability of negative states to take over our mind again in the future. By changing the station, we prepare the ground for positive mental states to become our default mode of being. The "half-full glass" is not far away. We do not have to look for it, or go somewhere else to find it. In fact, it is the same glass as the other one. We are not changing the glass, we are changing only the way we see it.

If you remember to do this consistently all day, day after day, negative thoughts, like thoughts that fuel depression, will slowly be transformed. Negative mental states also fuel family and workplace disputes. By practicing right diligence, you are tackling some of the root causes of difficult relationships as well as sleep difficulties.

the garden of the mind

> You cannot prevent the birds of sadness from flying overhead,
> but you can prevent them from roosting in your hair.
>
> —SWEDISH PROVERB

Another way to practice right diligence is to imagine yourself as a gardener. The garden you are tending is the garden of your mind. Is it a bare patch of ground? Is it overgrown with weeds and thorns? Start by cultivating a corner with beautiful flowers of joy and peace. Cultivate the flowers of gratitude. When you are in your garden, you can go to that corner so you can enjoy those nourishing flowers and take care of them. As you do so, they will grow and spread till more of the garden will be a pleasant place.

Just remember, though: A garden is not made in one day. And a garden is never finished.

ethical behavior for better sleep?

A clear conscience is a precious possession. Some people are aware of this, and are scrupulous about acting in accordance with the dictates of their conscience. They do not let greed for more power, more money, or more sex take over their mind and determine their actions. They are the lucky ones, because like everyone else, they will be alone with their conscience at night, and they will have one less thing to keep them awake.

Some others, like Macbeth and Lady Macbeth as portrayed in Shakespeare's play, discover the importance of ethical behavior only when they transgress its boundaries. "You don't know what you got till it's gone," as the saying goes. You can run away from bandits, but you cannot run away from yourself.

When I was traveling in Peru recently, a cabdriver asked me where I was from. This is a standard question for all gringos, but I like to turn it around, so I asked him the same question. We were in Lima, but he was from Cuzco. "Quechua," he said, and added, "Do not steal, do not lie, do not be dishonest. We have a moral code."

I looked at him, and saw a peaceful man. I was impressed that his moral code was on his mind and on the tip of his tongue, not somewhere on the shelf. Ethics has a bearing on everything we do. In his case, every time he quotes a price for a ride (there are no meters in Peruvian taxis), every time he scrambles for clients, and every evening as he does his accounting, his moral code can guide his actions. I got a feeling of oneness and simplicity from him. I felt that his moral code made life easier for him, both during the day, and at night when it was time to sleep.

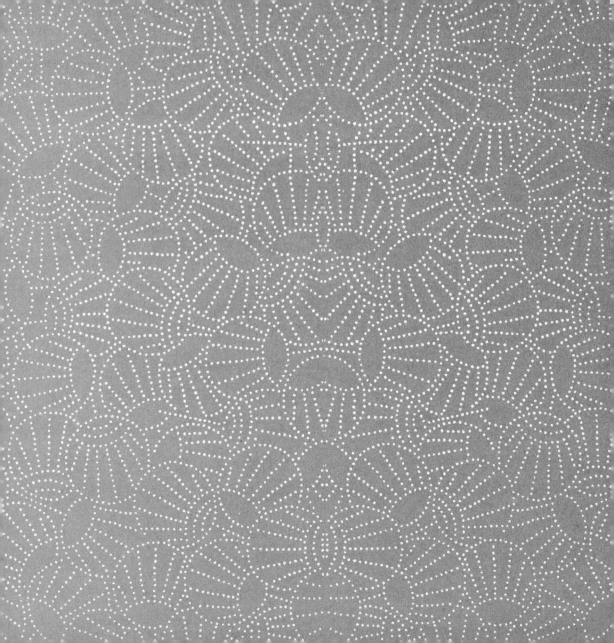

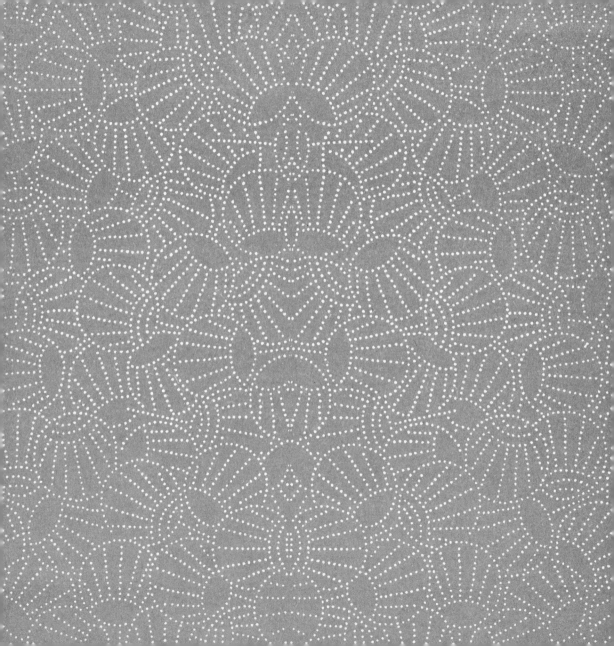

CHAPTER FIVE

The Conscious Mind and Sleep

t is the unconscious mind that does sleep. The conscious mind *prepares* us for sleep. It creates the physical conditions, does the bathroom routine, gets into bedclothes, turns off the light, and so on, but it has no clue about how to do sleep. The practice of mindfulness meditation gives us the tools to go one more step toward creating the conditions. With mindfulness meditation, we learn to create the *mental* conditions. We can prepare the *mind* for sleep.

Notice that as soon as we say, "I cannot go to sleep," we create two "I's": the "I" who wants to go to sleep but can't, and the "I" who knows how to do it but also can't, because the conditions are not right—or because the conscious mind gets in the way despite its best intentions. When a car runs smoothly, we do not have to bother with what is under the hood. But we look under the hood when it gives us problems. Looking at the way these two "I's" interact is like looking under the hood.

We do not have to make up theories and write books about how the right hand and the left hand should work together. In a peaceful person, the two minds work harmoniously and seamlessly, and they cooperate, as the right hand and the left hand cooperate when we eat or prepare a meal. The conscious mind turns off the light, and the unconscious mind does sleep, each doing its job at the right time according to its field of competence. We "just do it," as a popular slogan says. But when peace is not there, nothing seems to work. Just look at those parts of the world where there is conflict. The two sides do not listen to each other. They do not accept each other. They treat each other unkindly. They do not cooperate. These negative factors are also present in a person when there is inner conflict.

peace

I learned the full meaning of the word *peace* from Thich Nhat Hanh. He has explored the whole gamut of the meaning of that word, from the political arena, to peace in relationships and, most important, to inner peace. His sayings, written in his inimitable calligraphy, decorate my walls:

"Peace Is Every Breath." "Peace in Oneself, Peace in the World." "Peace Is Every Step."

"Peace Is Every Step" is also the title of one of his poems. I have set it to music, and do not tire of singing it to myself or in groups: *Peace is every step. It turns the endless path to joy.*

Inner peace comes when the different facets of our personality are in harmony. Like the proverbial pebble in the moccasin that tires us out more than the miles we walk, when we are conflicted about what we are doing, that inner conflict makes our task more exhausting. In contrast, inner peace turns the endless path of our life into joy.

The Persian poet Rumi comments on this point in the following lines:

> If we are not together in the heart, what's the point?
> When body and soul are not dancing,
> There is no pleasure in colorful clothing.

our two minds at play

It has been an adventure, first to be aware of the two or more "I's" that inhabit me, and then to reconcile their voices. I had to do this often while I recently learned to play the guitar as an adult. During the process of learning, my conscious mind was often the taskmaster. It would say things like, "Now you have to learn this chord and practice strumming." And my fingers, two hands, and parts of my brain would keep doing this task over and over again until it became *automatic*, meaning that my unconscious mind had finally learned to do it. Then, the conscious mind would set up another task.

The conscious mind acted as the adult or the more mature partner. The unconscious mind, on the other hand, could be childlike and could easily get discouraged: "Oh, this is impossible—it feels so awkward, and my fingers hurt." The conscious mind would then be a caring and wise adult: "Okay, I guess you have done enough for today. Take a break, and try again tomorrow. It will feel a little bit easier each time; you will see."

The elements of conflict are there, but the elements of peace are there as well: two sides are listening to each other. There is acceptance and adjustment. If the unconscious, childlike aspect ruled the roost, the conscious mind would capitulate, and I would give up trying to learn to play the guitar. If, on the other hand, the conscious taskmaster did not listen to the other side and pushed harder, the fun might go out of the project, or worse, some injury might happen. It is not unusual for people who push themselves beyond the point of endurance to develop injuries like carpal tunnel syndrome or tennis elbow. Can one also injure oneself while trying too hard to go to sleep? Yes, people do, with alcohol, "nightcaps," painkillers, and other addictive substances. In 2009, Michael Jackson tragically died in his search for sleep.

"Do not turn yourself into a battlefield," Thich Nhat Hanh often reminds us. Indeed, some people get upset at themselves when they have sleep difficulties. This irritation does not make sleep easier. The way of mindfulness meditation is a gentle one. With each breath we come home to ourselves. If there is pain inside, we listen, acknowledge, and hold the pain, as a mother holds her crying baby in her arms. This is a compassionate gesture, and brings comfort.

CHAPTER SIX

Mindfulness Practice

from camel to high-flying bird

The following two quotations from Rumi illustrate the difference between two modes of thinking. In the first one, the thinker is a slave to his thinking and does not question the authority of his thoughts. He is ruled by his thoughts:

Your thinking is like a camel driver,
and if you are the camel,
it drives you in every direction under its bitter control.

The second one shows a feeling of perspective and choice. The thinker remains in control, not the thoughts:

> At times, I give myself up to thought purposefully:
> But when I choose
> I spring up from those under its sway.

This is also the difference mindfulness makes. There is no wholesale rejection of thinking, no throwing out the baby with the bathwater. But the thinker is able to see her thoughts for what they are: just thoughts. With the perspective that a little distance gives, she can evaluate their appropriateness. She can consider whether they are emotion driven or objective, vengeful or loving. She is in a position to consider whether following her thoughts would bring happiness or misery.

Thoughts can loom large, like a huge balloon. But the pinprick of mindfulness can deflate this huge balloon and enable us to see it for what it is: a small piece of rubber. In the imagery of Rumi, it can turn the camel driver into a small insect, and the camel into a high-flying bird:

> I am like a high-flying bird
> And thought is a gnat:
> How should a gnat overpower me?

This perspective is precious. Thoughts can drive us to suicide or allow us to write sublime poetry; they can push us to declare war or to seek peace. Without mindfulness, following our thoughts indiscriminately can be a little bit like playing Russian roulette.

mindfulness and sleep

Matthew Syed is the author of *Bounce: The Myth of Talent and the Power of Practice*. In a BBC article about his work, he writes that when we are under stress, "Instead of using the subconscious part of the brain, which is the most efficient way to deliver a familiar skill (like talking, walking or remembering a math formula during an A-level), we use the conscious part. And this is when it all goes wrong." When that happens, we get tongue-tied, we freeze, we choke, and we do not do well.

The competence of sleep also lies in the unconscious, and when she is under stress, a highly skilled and educated adult may find that sleep eludes her. The irony is, of course, that the ability to sleep is available to a simple baby! The stressed adult wants to sleep so badly that this desire is getting in the way. It is making her try to manage sleep consciously instead of gently abandoning herself to the unconscious mind.

There is something about stress that makes us want to control things. Mindfulness is awareness of this as well as of our stress and our desires. It is a state of mind that brings freedom and peace. As we become aware that our attachment to control does not bring positive results, it is easier to let go. However, when we are stressed, letting go may be the last thing on our mind—it may go against the grain of the moment. The power of mindfulness can overcome that and make sleep possible.

mindfulness is a verb

As a practice, mindfulness is a verb disguised as a noun. It is not a state we achieve once and for all. It is something we practice with each breath. When we walk, balance is not something we achieve once and for all. It is something we find with each step. Our thinking is a bit like gravity—it pulls us out of balance all the time. Mindfulness allows us to find a balance between thinking and feeling as we return to the here and now over and over again.

> Mindfulness gives us the ability to bring our understanding, knowledge, and inspiration to bear upon this, and every moment of our life.

Our default mode of thinking is the survival mode. In the survival mode, our field of vision is contracted, and the larger picture is forgotten. This pits parent against child, spouse against spouse, and coworkers against each other.

"You are either for us, or against us," as George W. Bush once put it. However, in nature every being takes care of itself, *and also* fits into an ecological whole. There is harmony as well as strife. This is the larger picture. It is a picture of wholeness and interdependence.

impatience

Mind and body go at different speeds. The mind is quick. You think of a place, like the shopping mall, and you are already mentally there.

But the body is slow. It is still here.

Body and mind get separated again and again every time we get impatient, as may happen while we are waiting in line, or as we are getting a young child dressed to go out. In order to change old habits, we need a plan, and we need to stick to that plan for a certain length of time. This is like rehab.

no destination

No Destination is the title of Satish Kumar's autobiography. As a young man, Kumar undertook an eight-thousand-mile peace pilgrimage, walking from India to America without any money, through mountains, deserts, storms, and snow, in order to deliver a peace message to the nuclear capitals of the world. This trip definitely had a purpose, and Kumar was well acquainted with purposes and destinations. I was inspired by his book, but intrigued by its title. Why was it called *No Destination*?

I had a clue as I listened to Thich Nhat Hanh teaching walking meditation at Plum Village (I am quoting from memory): "You are going over there to look at that flower. That is your goal. But do not sacrifice the means for the goal. Every moment of your life is precious. The time you spend walking towards the flower is as precious as the moment when you arrive there. Enjoy every moment. Arrive in the here and now with every step."

Indeed, if the destination is all that counts, there are more efficient ways of going from India to the United States. In the larger context of an autobiography, life is a journey, a journey without destination. Either we enjoy every step of the journey, or we have missed out.

At another time, Thich Nhat Hanh introduced a period of walking meditation with the words, "It is as if you have an armful of precious jewels. And you throw away all these jewels." It took me a while to understand the full significance of his words, and of the sweeping gesture of scattering jewels to the ground that he made while he spoke. This is how we live. Each moment of our life is a precious jewel. But, fixated on where we are going, we are oblivious to the beauty around us, the beauty of life.

To be successful in learning mindfulness meditation techniques, we need to accept going at a slower speed so that there is time for overcoming old habits. Living in mindfulness means savoring each moment. In order to do that, we need to overcome the mind's habit of wanting to jump to the future. The same mental habit that makes us jump ahead to tomorrow and creates worry also makes us impatient. The mind needs to slow down in order to enjoy the present moment. It needs to learn to get out of the way sometimes.

Do not identify with the part of you that is impatient. Impatience is not the solution; it is part of the problem. MMT is not a physical operation like liposuction that will produce instant results. It is not a chemical agent like anesthesia that will knock you out. I have seen that many people do not want to accept that. They may come to mindfulness meditation after years of trying other approaches that have failed to deliver results. They have waited years before, but now they want instant results from MMT.

You need to forget about your expectations, about the end result, and enjoy the path for a while. Enjoy the journey, and take your mind off the destination. Get into the meditation exercises. Enjoy the peace and relaxation they provide. Enlightenment is available only in the present moment. Be in the moment and savor it. Paradoxically, only then will the results you seek begin to happen.

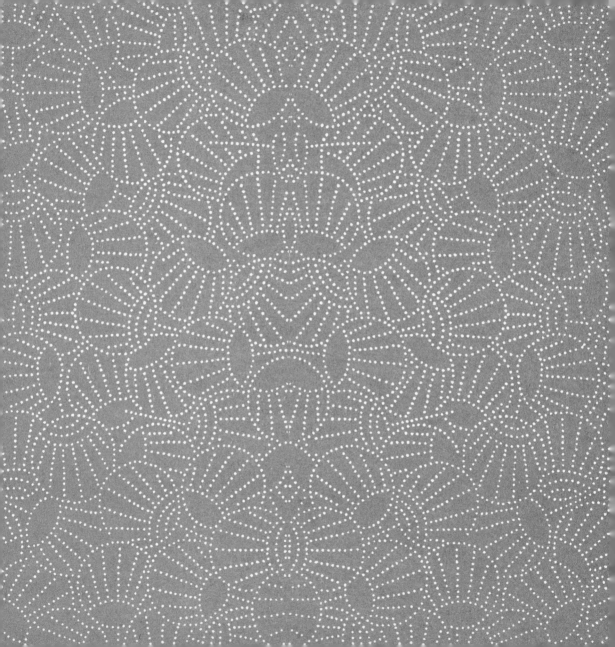

CHAPTER SEVEN

Meditation and Action

why we need meditation

We need an intermediate time between a day of action and a night of rest.

   The time we set aside for meditation is just such a time. It is a time when we are alone with ourselves—it is a time for healing. Unless we set aside such a time, sleep time is left as the only moment when we are *looking inward, quiet* and *undistracted*. These three conditions are also the conditions for meditation. If we do not set aside a time for meditation, sleep time doubles as reflection time. But without the qualities that make meditation such a healing activity, reflection may plunge us into rumination, regrets, worries, and keep us awake. In meditation we first quiet the mind by getting in touch with our breath. This allows us to see things from a wider perspective. We practice freedom. You will notice this approach in the guided meditations in this book.

During the day, there are all kinds of distractions to take our mind off important issues. But once the light is off at night, the distractions end, and we are left alone with our problems. In a way, this is as it should be. We are not in a position to contemplate relationships or career issues while the phone is ringing, clients are waiting, or we are dodging other cars on the road. However, the unconscious mind knows these things are important, and brings them up when it gets the chance, and the only chance it gets may be at bedtime. We have failed to provide time to look deeply into important issues. Our agenda has failed to make space for some intermediate time between go, go, go and sleep—some time to be a human *being* after a day of human *doing*.

The effect of this in our waking life is that only the first few items on our to-do list get done—the urgent ones, not necessarily the important ones. The effect on our sleeping is that the rest of the list may hit us with full force when we turn the lights off.

What usually passes for relaxation does not address this issue. Neither does watching TV, reading a novel, or sipping beer. They will only postpone things that need attention. The issues will still be there when we turn the lights off. Meditation is a chance to see things deeply, to go beyond the surface. Mindfulness meditation is about living our own life more fully, more gracefully, and with inspiration. Far from being separate from life and action, the fruits of meditation are in how we live, in how we do ordinary as well as extraordinary things.

The bronze statue that is forever sitting does not convey the full scope of Buddha's life. Buddha's life had action as well as contemplation. He did not only sit on his insights, he also acted on them. He started with leaving behind the maelstrom of courtly life that had become meaningless for him, and embarked on a new life of self-discovery and self-realization. As head of a large community, he had responsibility for 1,250 monks (if you have your hands full with your family of just three or four, just multiply the number of problems you have by a few hundred to get a feel for the responsibilities he had). He was also advising kings, businessmen, and common folk, and walking all over India to spread the practice of the Dharma. He was not a hermit.

meditation and action go together

When meditation becomes a part of our life, transformation and change are not far behind. We embark on this path by first calming the mind and paying attention to the breath.

The usual state of our mind may be like downtown traffic, with many thoughts coming and going every which way. Once the traffic has calmed down, we watch and listen. If there is a concern just below the surface of the mind, we listen to that. If there is discomfort about something, we note that. Then, we might decide to make some changes, or take some kind of action if that is appropriate.

Meditation is not only about sitting. Meditation is not about awakening to Buddha's life. He lived twenty-six centuries ago, in quite different circumstances. Meditation is about awakening to our own life. One cannot separate meditation from action. Either we make changes inspired by our meditation, or we are forever stuck at the same place, forever experiencing the same regrets or worries, forever being kept awake at night. If you are in an abusive relationship, just sitting will not fix that. Sitting may make things clear, it may give you courage, and it may help you find inspired solutions. But then you have to get up and do whatever else is necessary to bring your life more in line with your insights.

Looking at meditation this way may give you a different perspective on it. It may help you to see it as a proactive practice, instead of only a passive practice.

right action

Meditation makes appropriate action possible. With the mind and emotions calmed, and aware of our connection and love for all beings, we can act from a peaceful place. This kind of action is beneficial for us as well as others. It is not a knee-jerk sort of reaction. It comes from a deeper place, and is healing for all concerned.

There are problems with acting emotionally, acting in a state of panic, or acting out of greed or egoism. If we act out of those places, we may soon be caught in regret, the problems may still persist, and cycles of inappropriate action and regret may continue to haunt us and keep us awake at night.

By the way, sometimes doing nothing is the appropriate action. But when we choose to do nothing, it is not because we are afraid to act, or because we are confused. Rather it is because we have seen that doing nothing is the "right action" given the circumstances.

attitude

People stay up all the time. They stay up to watch a show on television, they stay up to continue to drink at a bar, they stay up to talk to friends, and they stay up to read or to work on their computer. Their thoughts around this kind of voluntary sleep deprivation are something like:

"I'm having fun. I like to do this. It is my choice."

It is getting up in the morning that is often more problematic.

Becoming aware of our attitudes is an important part of mindfulness practice, because the "I didn't get enough" feeling itself can be a source of anxiety, and not only with regard to sleep. People who feel they did not get enough (money, sex, love, whatever) make themselves unhappy. And some people always feel that they should get more of whatever it is, including sleep.

Look deeply into your attitudes: Do you feel that your day is out of control, that it does not belong to you? Could it be that this is why you have a need to stay up late, so you can finally do the things that you enjoy? If so, sleep deprivation is not so much the problem. Maybe you have a satisfaction deprivation.

Mindfulness meditation is a wonderful tool for making each day, each moment of our life count.

Paradoxically, this is achieved not by doing more, but by doing less.

We may feel that we need to do the things that have to be done faster so that we have time for doing more things. Mindfulness practice goes the other way. I may need to go to the store to get a carton of milk. The way to make the experience more satisfying is not doing it as fast as possible while thinking of other things, but to enjoy the walk or the bike ride to the store by paying attention. This way, we make each moment count. We are not sacrificing the *means* for the *goal*. Otherwise, our day becomes a series of dry chores. When night comes, we may feel that we haven't lived.

> Life is so short, we should all move more slowly.   —Thich Nhat Hanh

As each day becomes more beautiful and satisfying, it becomes easier to let go. The day is no longer incomplete. We did not simply run out of time. The day is full and done, and now it is time for sleep. We have lived this day fully, and we are no longer hungry for more. This is like the feeling after a satisfying meal.

focusing on the experience, not on the one having the experience

> At last, the sky is empty
> No birds, no clouds
> The mountain and I sit together
> Till there is only the mountain.
>
> —LI PO (701–762)

When the self is in the picture, it is easy to wrap a drama around it. If you are having a sleep difficulty, the drama might go something like, "It is terrible that I do not sleep enough." "Poor me, I'm going to feel sleepy all day tomorrow." "Am I going to have this problem all my life?" "Why me?" and so on. This drama does not help. Indeed, with time, it can itself become an impediment to sleep as we alternately worry about the fate of this "I" and become irritated with it.

Getting ourselves out of the way is a good way to end the drama. We can do this by focusing on only what we are experiencing. If you have some pain due to a health condition, do not embroider stories around the pain, or around the person who has the pain. Just staying with the raw sensation, you may discover that pain itself isn't as bad as the stories we make up around it. If your experience is "Wide Awake," so be it. Do not weave stories around the wide-awake person. Relax and use this gift of time wisely. If you play your cards right, you may have time for some sleep later.

learning to live with discomfort

We are always something: we are either tired, or sleepy, or bored, or impatient, or thirsty, or hungry, or angry, or sexually excited, or worried, or frustrated . . . the list of all the things we can be is long. We will stop being this or that only when we are dead. Think about this when you wish for that moment when nothing bothers you. Being a little bit uncomfortable is part of life. The Buddhist teacher Pema Chödrön addresses this subject in her book *The Wisdom of No Escape.*

This wisdom comes when we accept inconveniences and stop wishing for perfect bliss. Then, perfect bliss may come, not as the absence of disturbing feelings or mental states, but as a result of a change of attitude. It is not the absence of discomfort or whatever it is, but our attitude toward it that makes the difference. The discomfort might still be there, but it does not fill the whole of our mental space.

Once in a group session, Michael, a retired teacher, was describing his unhappy weekends: "My neighbor ties the dog outside, and leaves for the weekend. The dog is always barking all weekend. I cannot enjoy my own backyard."

Alice asked him a pointed question: "What bothers you more: the dog, or your own irritation?"

This exchange has stayed with me, because what bothers us, and keeps us awake, is our own response to a situation as much or more than the situation itself. Just to know this fact is helpful, because we are not going to be able to solve every single problem, and eliminate every barking dog. Yet, accepting all inconveniences is not the complete solution either. I think the Serenity Prayer strikes a good balance:

> God grant me the serenity to accept the things I cannot change;
> Courage to change the things I can;
> and wisdom to know the difference.

However, as far as sleep is concerned, skewing the balance in favor of acceptance is often the wiser choice. I relearned this truth recently in a noisy hotel in Lima, Peru. I had booked this hotel online for an overnight stay because it was close to the airport. However, it turned out to be a noisy place. I did well for a while and continued sleeping through various disturbances. Then another burst of noise occurred, close to my door. I remember thinking in my sleep that if I opened the door and asked them to be quiet, everything would be all right for the rest of the night, so I got up, and did it. It turned out to be the wrong choice. I had not anticipated that getting up to go to the door would wake me up completely, and asking the people outside to be quiet would turn a small irritation into a bigger one. I ended up staying awake for a while after that. As I did, I also noticed that as the night stretched into the wee hours, the noises died of their own accord.

talk back to your mind

Indeed, how do we know when to accept a discomfort, and when to act to change it? Accepting a discomfort goes against the popular wisdom that says, "Listen to your body." Yet our bodies are often saying things like, "Have another helping—this food is so good," or, "Have another beer." This is how many of us become overweight or inebriated—by listening to ourselves. When the alarm rings in the morning, the body says, "Sleep some more. It feels so good." Yet, the night before, the same body might have been saying, "Stay up some more. It feels so good." How do we know when to listen and when to talk back?

The Buddha addressed this question more than once. His answer is that happiness does not come through torturing the body, and not through indulging it. It is the middle way that brings freedom. It is clear that many of us have not found this middle way in regard to food.

There is also a middle way between conscientiousness and relaxation. We cannot wait until all the problems have been solved and everything on our to-do list has been accomplished before we allow ourselves to fall asleep. At a certain point, we need to stop listening to the mind that says, "You did not do enough," and start talking back. We can say, "Thank you, mind. Thank you." We can even repeat this like a mantra.

being gentle with yourself

If you feel angry with yourself because you cannot sleep or for some other reason, just remember that the person you are angry with is also yourself. You will not find contentment or sleep by beating on yourself. The part of you that receives the beating will be unhappy. *You* will be unhappy. That will not make sleep any easier.

"Anxiety may manifest as anxiety about sleep. Many anxious adults were anxious as children. Dr. Bonnie Zucker, in her book *Anxiety-Free Kids*, quotes research showing that 20 percent of children and adolescents suffer from anxiety, and that many anxious children become anxious adults. Some authors estimate the percentage of childhood anxiety that persists into adulthood to be as high as 90 percent. Unlike disruptive or aggressive behavior for which a child's teacher may call home, childhood anxiety is often not a problem in the classroom, and may go unnoticed and untreated. Marc Weissbluth, M.D., gives a scary warning in his book *Healthy Sleep Habits, Happy Child*: "If your child does not learn to sleep well, he may become an incurable adult insomniac, chronically disabled from sleepiness and dependent on sleeping pills." The roots of our discomfort with sleep may lie deep, and we may need to look just as deeply to find them.

turning disturbances into lullabies

The same person who may be complaining about being kept up by noise might choose to go to sleep with the radio on. The difference is that she is not fighting with the radio as she may have been fighting with "the noise." The same noise that disturbs one sleeper may have no effect on another. It all depends on our attitude and the stories we tell ourselves.

Some amount of noise and distraction may indeed be beneficial for going to sleep: people fall asleep while driving, and even, according to some recent news reports, while working as a subway ticket vendor or an air traffic controller. Any distraction takes one's mind off thinking, and may facilitate sleep.

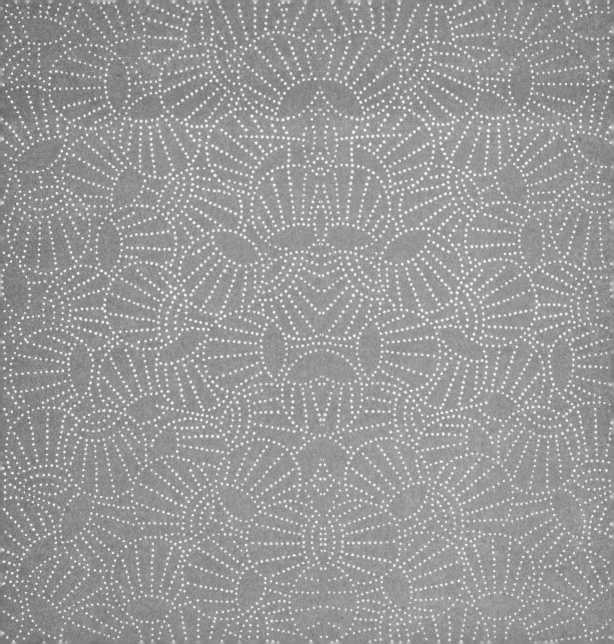

PART TWO

Guided Meditation Exercises— Seven Weeks Toward Mastering Mindfulness Meditation

introduction to exercises

Many resolutions fall by the wayside because we forget about them. Others are abandoned because we lack information: it is not enough to know *where* we want to go—we also need to know *how* to get there. And sometimes we may run out of steam along the way: inspiration is the steam that propels us forward. Yesterday's inspiration may not be enough to keep us going today. We need fresh inspiration every day.

This section of the book contains passages that you need to read before a meditation period. To get results, your practice needs to be nourished and renewed with short readings, preferably *every* time you sit down to meditate.

> Reading before a period of meditation has three purposes:
> Inform, Remind, and Inspire.

You need information to keep you on track. Information guides you during your meditation practice. It also has to be readily available, at your fingertips. You read a passage once for information. You read it again and again for keeping it fresh in your memory.

Inspiration is just as important as information. You come to meditation with a mind full of other things. If you sit in this state, you may find that those things that occupied your mind before you sat will continue to run through your mind while you sit. You may look as if you are meditating, but you may not be concentrating wholeheartedly. After a few sessions like this, you may find the experience unsatisfactory, and stop trying.

If you have only fifteen minutes to spare for meditation practice today, divide that time between reading and sitting. Take five minutes to read an appropriate text first, and then sit for ten minutes. You may go further than if you just plunked yourself down on a cushion cold.

Inspiration is different from information. Inspiration reminds you why you are doing what you are doing, while information tells you how to do it. Inspiration is like a vow, or a resolution. It gives you direction and purpose. You need it to keep going. Often, when it is time to sit, you may be far away in your mind from sitting. Inspiration will bring you to the vicinity, bring you close, to the threshold of meditation. It will remind you once again why you are doing this. Then your practice will be purposeful and wholehearted.

> You need all three:
> Inspiration
> Information
> Practice

Practice makes your vows and resolutions a reality. Meditation is a skill, like learning to play the piano. If you learn only one song, you will soon get tired of playing it. Your meditation needs to evolve and develop to keep you practicing. That's why there are seven different meditations in this book: to keep your interest level up.

Each of the following exercises comes with an introduction as well as a short text in italics to read before you start meditating. You might like to read that text aloud. That way, you will have an auditory as well as a visual memory of it. After reading a text, look it over again to see what you remember. It is what you remember that counts.

Now put the book away, and practice each phrase, instruction, or image that you remember for five breaths (one breath consists of an in breath and an out breath). You can do this by mentally repeating the phrase, visualizing the image, or following the instruction.

You can count the five breaths with your fingers. This is work: it takes concentration to stay on track. When you run out of things you remember, you can continue to sit a little longer, or stop. You can also read the text once more and meditate again.

The first time you do this, your session may take only ten minutes: five for reading, and perhaps a minute each on five instructions that you remember. When you do the same meditation once more or the next day, it may take a little bit longer, because you will probably remember a few more instructions. What is important is that you keep up the awareness of breath—without this awareness, you may find yourself daydreaming.

As your meditation periods get longer, you may find yourself "glowing." I do not know how else to describe the wonderful feeling of well-being that meditation brings. You can bask in that glow as long as you keep concentrating on the breath.

A word about what to do with the eyes. When I am meditating, my eyes are almost closed, like venetian blinds that are pulled down, but not tightly all the way, so that a little light is still showing at the bottom. I do not try to focus on or look at anything. Usually, all that gets through is a little bit of light and a little bit of color. This works for me. If I close my eyes all the way, I am more likely to be in my thoughts. On the other hand, opening them all the way can be distracting.

We cannot close down the other senses, and we cannot close down the mind. Our ears are always open, even when we are not listening actively or analyzing what we hear. Similarly, during meditation the eyes are not closed tight, but they are not looking at anything or focusing on anything specific either.

I suggest that you stay with one exercise each week, and do it for seven days. After you have gone through all the exercises, if you want a review or if you want more practice, you can switch to doing a different exercise each day of the week. However, feel free to personalize your practice regimen and make changes.

The same goes for when you do these exercises and where you do them.

The obvious choice would be to do them before going to sleep and in your bedroom. But we all have different sleeping arrangements and different bedroom furniture. Experiment with different routines until you find what works for you.

> If your problem is waking up in the early hours of the morning,
> you can switch to doing the exercises at that time.

I recommend a sitting posture. Personally, I find it difficult to meditate lying down. Meditation requires both relaxation *and* concentration. While the lying-down posture is good for relaxation, it is not so good for concentration. Experiment to see if you agree.

If you are sitting on the floor, the sitting posture requires that the buttocks be elevated a bit. Otherwise it is easy to slouch. You need to sit on a hard cushion or on a meditation bench.

If you are sitting on a chair, keep both feet flat on the ground. On the bed or in the bed, just pop a pillow under your buttocks.

Keep the hands crossed on your lap. It helps if the hands are in contact with the belly, which is expanding and contracting as you breathe. That contact point gives you another source of feedback on your breath.

Week One—Calming the Mind

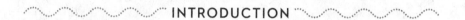

Some people think that the purpose of meditation is to stop the mind. They sit, and they try. Soon they get into a fight with their mind, a fight that they lose. Frustrated, they give up. Do you recognize yourself in this scenario?

Calming the mind is a more appropriate goal, and a good way to do it is by paying attention to the breath. When we are daydreaming, the breath follows the rhythm of our thoughts. That rhythm can be irregular, because we are going from thought to thought, from one thing to another. As we continue to follow the *breath* instead of our thoughts, the breath gets into a steady, regular rhythm.

> Meditation is not the same thing as daydreaming.

Usually we follow our thoughts without any attention to the breath. Here, we reverse that—we follow our breath. At the beginning, we treat our thoughts a little bit like the way we treat the radio in the background. As we do other things, we are aware that the radio is playing, but we do not follow it actively. For example, when the announcer says, "Go and buy that car right now, because it is so amazing," we do not drop everything and rush out to buy it. We have learned to take an attitude of sophisticated detachment with regard to the radio. Now we cultivate the same detached attitude toward our thoughts.

Our work in meditation right now is concentrating on the breath. This means staying with the breath and the sensations of the breath continuously. I don't know if you have ever followed a *single* breath from end to end, and paid attention to all the sensations that occur. One single breath can make you aware of your posture, of how tight your belt is, and of any tension in your abdominal muscles.

> If you are a chest breather, please take a few minutes to read the
> section on diaphragmatic breathing at the end of the book, and
> do the simple exercises that will get you started. To find out how
> you breathe, put your hand on your abdomen and breathe in.
> Your hand should go out as you breathe in.

The breath is like a swing in the playground. As you breathe in, first it accelerates. Then it slows down near the end. Then it comes to an unstable stop and starts going again in the other direction. The speed is always changing. To notice all this, you need not only awareness, but also concentration. You need to concentrate so that you are not only aware during brief moments of this cycle, but you are continuously aware of it during the whole cycle, cycle after cycle.

> I Can Feel My Breath in a Number of Ways:
>
> I can feel it in my diaphragm.
>
> I can feel my clothes adjusting as my diaphragm changes shape.
>
> I can feel the rush of air in my nostrils.
>
> I can also feel a coolness around my nostrils as I breathe in.

If you have trouble noticing that last item, put your finger horizontally against your nostrils for a few seconds. You will feel the change of temperature as you breathe in and out.

By concentrating on the breath, we are offering the mind something other than thoughts to chew on. This works better than fighting with it to get it to slow down.

Within a few minutes, something different starts to happen: the breath finds its natural rhythm. In normal wakefulness, thoughts are zipping through the mind, and the breath is irregular and staccato. Now the breath follows a more regular rhythm, like that of the waves on the beach. Like the waves, the breath comes from somewhere we don't know. Then it goes inside, and gets lost, like the waves that get absorbed into the sand. Some of the water gets returned back to the ocean, but it is not exactly the same. Now it has cleaned the beach and is carrying back some debris and also the warmth of the sand with it. The breath has also just cleaned the body, and the out breath is warm and full of carbon dioxide. You can let yourself be guided by this mental imagery. Involve all your senses and now bask in the sunshine on that beach for a few minutes and enjoy the *whishsh* of the waves.

Another metaphor: What is happening in the mind at this point is also a little bit like the difference between city driving and long-distance driving. In city driving, there is much stopping and starting and emotions like impatience or irritation. When you settle into long-distance driving, all those calm down. The rhythm changes.

During this breathing exercise, you may find that, after a while, concentration comes naturally. At the beginning, concentration required effort. Now this natural rhythm of the breath takes over. You may feel like a seagull that has got off the ground with much flapping of the wings and is now soaring effortlessly with the wind. Enjoy riding the winds of breath. Let a smile of contentment penetrate your heart.

Thoughts lose their urgency at this stage.

You have arrived at the meditative state. This state is itself as restful as sleep, and according to some, even more so. You can enjoy it as long as you like, or as long as it lasts.

> Read this and other meditation texts slowly, with a short pause
> between instructions.

The past has already gone and the future is yet to come.
I am concentrating on being peaceful, happy, and free in this present moment.

•

Now I'm concentrating on being aware of each breath.
My attention on the breath is continuous.
I follow the breath as it begins, and my abdomen starts to expand.
I continue to pay attention as my abdomen rises and falls with each breath,
like a child going high and low on a swing.

•

Like a swing, my breath slows down at each end.
I follow it all the way as it slows down, and starts again.

•

I embrace my breath with all my care and attention,
like a mother holds her baby.
I do not drop the baby.
Thoughts stay in the background.

•

I enjoy the rhythmic rise and fall of my abdomen;
I enjoy staying in the here and the now.
I have stopped running forward and backward.

•

My mind keeps producing thoughts; that is its nature.
I do not follow the thoughts.
I concentrate on my breath.

•

I'm comfortable and at ease.
With each breath, I let go of tension somewhere in my body and mind.

•

I'm aware that thoughts can bring tension to my face.
With each breath, I relax my face muscles and smile.

•

There are sensations in my body, I accept them. I am aware of my posture.
I am aware of the rush of air around my nostrils as I breathe in.

•

If there are sounds, I do not react to them.
I just notice them and let them go.
I continue to enjoy my breathing peacefully.

•

A river of feelings and thoughts is flowing, but I am not drowning in it.

The concentration on the breath is like the anchor that
prevents the boat from drifting.

•

Focusing on my breath keeps me from getting lost in thought.
I notice sounds and skin sensations without reacting to them.

•

I smile at disturbances such as memories, little itches, and noises.
Smiling relaxes me. I feel content.

•

With each breath I arrive in the here and the now—
I'm sitting upright, breathing comfortably.

•

My mind is peaceful, my body free of tension.
I am calm and rested.
I feel free. I feel at home.

Week Two—Taming the Mind

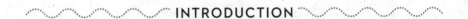 **INTRODUCTION**

Now that the mind is calmer, it is ready to be tamed.

Thinking is not our enemy. We owe most of our successes in life to it. But it can be our enemy when it is automatic, repetitive, based on old habits, and constantly running forward to the future or backward to the past. Such thinking does not bring benefits. On the contrary, it prevents us from being present during the day, and it may prevent us from sleeping at night. The remedy is not to stop all mental activity. This is not a realistic goal. The heart will continue to beat, the stomach will continue to digest, and the mind will continue to be active whether we want it to or not.

In mindfulness practice, we give the mind something else to do, something other than thinking. We ask it to follow the breath and to be aware of all the sensations of our bodies, of our posture, of comfort or discomfort in our legs and feet, and heat and cold in different body parts. We put our attention on what we are feeling rather than what we are thinking, and for the moment consider our thinking as some kind of background noise.

In a later stage, we will take another approach and practice awareness of states of mind so that we can become more conscious of our mental habits. But at this stage, our focus is on being able to overcome the strong pull of our thinking mind. It is a slippery situation: the attention keeps slipping back to our thoughts. We need to keep bringing it back gently to our body and to our breath, with each breath. When you experience this slipperiness, don't think that you are doing something wrong or that your meditation is not working. This is how meditation goes at the beginning, and also for some time after the beginning.

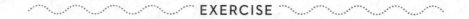 **EXERCISE**

*With each breath, I bring my attention from my thoughts
to what is happening in my body.
With each breath, I arrive from the world of thoughts to the world of the senses.*

·

*I am in the present moment when I concentrate on my breath
and on the flow of experience.*

·

*I focus just on the sensations themselves and not on the
person who is having these sensations.*

·

I focus on the sensations and not on my feelings about sensations.
For now, there's no good or bad, no judgments.

•

My senses take in the present moment.
I accept what comes in through my senses.

•

I accept the world as it is.
Breathing in and out, I remain in this warm world of acceptance.

•

Breathing in and out, I find contentment here and now.
I'm not struggling to want things to be otherwise.

•

Nothing to criticize, nothing to evaluate; those are thoughts.
Now I am just taking in what comes through my senses.

•

I count my blessings and send waves of contentment to
every part of my body.
My body is a miracle.

•

Thoughts come and go just like the noises around me.
I stay with my breath.

•

Breathing in and out, I stay open without striving.
I do not control the flow of insight. I only control my openness.

•

Is my mind free now?
I take one breath with freedom.
Then another.

•

Breathing in, I feel fresh.
Breathing out, I am still here.

While doing this exercise, read the text out loud slowly, and then start meditating. After a while, if you are happy with how your meditation is going, continue meditating. If you are running out of steam, go back and read the text out loud again, and try once more.

Week Three—Body Scan

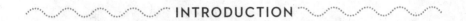

Some teachers start meditation training with the body scan. However, unless we address the magnetic pull our thinking has on us and calm the mind, we may find ourselves slipping into the thinking mode as we scan the body. Feel free to change the order of the exercises if it suits you better.

Also, many prefer doing the body scan in a lying-down position, because that position promotes a more complete relaxation. Feel free to do this exercise either lying down or sitting in the usual meditation pose. Personally, I find it difficult to concentrate in a lying-down position and am likely to lose track. If you lose track because you fall asleep, no problem. But if you lose track because you start thinking of other things, this could be counterproductive. If this happens, change your position and sit up.

The body scan has the purpose of focusing on different body parts and relaxing them consciously one by one.

Memory tip: We focus from the top down in the following order: Breath, Mind, Face, Neck and Shoulders, Abdomen, and Lower Body.

EXERCISE

Sitting comfortably, I let go of all tension.
I take five slow and deep breaths, concentrating on the
physical sensations of breathing,
on the rush of air in my nostrils as I breathe in, and on my expanding abdomen.
I am also aware of my belt or shifting clothes as my abdomen fills with air.
I keep my attention on the breath continuously through five breathing cycles:
in, slow down at the end, begin to exhale, slow down again,
brief pause, and start over.

·

With the next five breaths, I relax my mind.
Now, there is nothing to do and nowhere to go.
No obligations. I can just enjoy sitting, relaxing, and being myself.

·

The face is the mirror of the mind.
A peaceful face is the mirror of a peaceful mind.
My face reflects my inner smile.
I monitor my face muscle and my forehead, then my eyes and cheeks,
and then the muscles around my mouth and under my chin for five breaths.

·

I find a comfortable place for my chin that is neither too high nor too low.

With the next five breaths, I concentrate on my chin and my neck.
I make sure that my head is in alignment with my spine, and my neck is relaxed.

·

Going down farther, I concentrate on my shoulders and arms,
making sure that there is no tension in my shoulders.
My hands touch each other, and they also touch my abdomen.
With my hands I can feel my abdomen rising and falling.
I follow the peaceful rise and fall of my abdomen for the next five breaths.

·

In the meditation pose, the muscles in my back are engaged.
They keep me from slouching, so that there is room for
the breath in my abdomen.
I'm soft in the front, and hard in the back.
I breathe for five cycles, immobile in the back,
and moving rhythmically in the front.

·

I mentally follow the back muscles down toward my lower back.
The roots of my posture go all the way from the shoulders to my lower back.
My posture is steady, as the front and sides of my upper
body expand and contract with each breath.
My whole torso breathes.

·

With the next five breaths, I focus on the lower part of my body.
First, I focus on how the cushion, bench, or chair feels under my buttocks.
Am I well balanced?
If I need to make small adjustments for better balance
or comfort, I make them.

·

Next the legs. If there is some discomfort in the legs, I focus on it.
How does it actually feel?
I breathe in and out with awareness of that feeling.

·

For the next five breaths, I focus on my feet.
What are they resting on?
Is there a feeling of heat or cold on the feet?
Do both feet have the same feeling?
Where exactly is that feeling most intense? How do the ankles feel?

·

Finally, I feel the wholeness of my body from my head to my feet.
I feel how it all holds together as one body.

·

Now I listen. Is any part of my body or mind saying something?
Perhaps one foot is uncomfortable, and is complaining loudly.
Or the shoulders have tightened up. I let go. Then I listen again.

That last instruction of listening is important in order to be aware of where we are holding tension. It can be practiced often during the day. As we practice listening, we can take a load off our shoulders, or our chest.

Tension creeps up on us when we are thinking and not listening. Face muscles, abdomen, legs, and feet are all likely places that sometimes tense up. However, we are all different in where we hold tension. Once you become aware of where *you* tend to tense up, you can go directly to that place and relax the tension.

Taking some time to listen needs to be part of every meditation session. The instruction "smile" also means "relax face muscles." You can also post a LISTEN sign in a strategic spot around the house as a reminder. You will find that this reminder is not helpful only during meditation, but also all through the day.

Find a comfortable position while doing this exercise. However, "be comfortable" does not mean "slouch." In the meditation position, there is often some discomfort somewhere. Awareness and acceptance of this minimal discomfort is part of the practice.

A quick memory check: go from the top down, focusing on the Breath, Mind, Face, Neck and Shoulders, Abdomen, and Lower Body. This order is not important, but it makes remembering easier.

Week Four—Loving Kindness Meditation

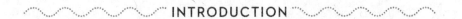 INTRODUCTION

It can be difficult to go to sleep if we are feeling angry. Angry thoughts can keep invading our mind, and get us all worked up. When we have strong feelings, it takes a lot of concentration to focus on the breath. Angry thoughts can break through our focus. At such times, loving kindness meditation can help. Loving kindness is the opposite of anger. Just like anger, it is also a mix of feelings and thoughts. A thought of compassion can be enough to interrupt a cascade of angry thoughts and bring us a sense of perspective.

I had occasion to put this in practice recently. Like many others, the lakeside town I live in, just west of Montreal, has been hit by a wave of graffiti. As I walked past a graceful, century-old building in the village, I noticed that the spacious chimneys on top of the building were now covered with fresh graffiti. I felt a wave of anger arising as I first saw the ugly black scrawls. Then I reflected on the need that these young men had for some kind of recognition. Somehow, that need has not been properly channeled by the school and the community. Indeed, just a year ago, three graffiti writers were killed by a train near here while they were writing their tags on an overpass in the middle of the night. Their need for recognition and achievement must have been quite intense, indeed, desperate. "Poor kids," I thought. "If this is their idea of recognition and achievement, their minds and hearts must be bleak indeed." My anger subsided.

I was not condoning graffiti as I let go of my anger. I still wished for some kind of deterrent or consequences for the perpetrators. This is not a plea for permissiveness. It is an acknowledgment that the ugly black scrawls are just the tip of the iceberg. Here, I am letting go of the graffiti writers, because my focus is on the transformation of anger. "A drop of compassion is enough to bring back spring on earth," Thich Nhat Hanh says. On this occasion, it was enough to bring back spring in my heart.

Loving kindness is an absence of ill will. It is a positive, friendly attitude, a wish for all beings to find joy and happiness in their lives. The many meanings of the word *love* can create confusion. Wanting other beings to be happy does not mean that we want to live with them. I do not want to live in a tigers' den or in a rabbit hole, although I love both those animals. I do not want to live with a smoker, although I wish smokers well. I do not even particularly want to live with a meat eater; my partner is a vegetarian like myself, and it simplifies things greatly. We shop and cook for each other.

What about people who commit murder and rape, or other kinds of unacceptable actions? This question comes up regularly in our groups when we are discussing loving kindness. My favorite answer is to point to the example of the Dalai Lama. He and the Tibetans have been wronged for a long time by the Chinese. If the Dalai Lama were angry at the Chinese, his heart would be quite an angry place indeed: there are a great many Chinese to be angry at. Instead, we all know what a kindhearted and jovial person he is. His secret? He makes a distinction between an action and the person who performs the action. As he explains in his book *Emotional Awareness,* an action can be quite unacceptable, and indeed hateful. But the person who performs the action can be seen as a victim of their own ignorance, greed, or attachment. In the case of the Chinese, they see the world through the colored glasses of communist dogma. Soldiers are under command and well indoctrinated. Each individual Chinese person involved in the tragedy of Tibet may be a victim of their misperceptions, of a sort of collective blindness. The Dalai Lama's attitude can be summed up as Hate the sin, but not the sinner.

Thich Nhat Hanh suggests another way of finding that drop of compassion for a difficult person: think of him when he was five years old and still vulnerable and beautiful. I have heard him suggest that to a young man who was having difficulty reconnecting with his father.

EXERCISE

Sitting comfortably, I take a few deep breaths.
I get in touch with any lingering feelings I have, and consciously replace them
with thoughts of goodwill.

•

I notice that there is a certain emotional tone that
comes up as I think of each person.
While the memory of certain persons makes me smile,
others make me tense up.

•

As I breathe in and out, I consciously substitute feelings of
kindness and friendliness toward each person
instead of this spontaneously appearing emotional tone.

•

I keep doing this over and over.
As an image or a name comes to mind,
I think of the person with warmth and kindness.
These feelings are mine. My feelings are not controlled by others.
I am responsible for my own feelings.

•

These kind and friendly feelings benefit me as well.
Ill will, anger, and grudges create stress.

·

I'm not playing favorites. I'm generous with my thoughts of goodwill.
Kindness is like sunshine. Everybody needs some.
The sun does not shine only on people who are perfect.
My kindness shines on each person, including myself.

·

I visualize myself as a five-year-old child, innocent and beautiful.
I have been that child.
I deserve my own love and kindness.
I deserve my own loving feelings now.

·

Many prisoners have been abused as children. They are victims.
They also need kindness. Kindness is medicine.
I do not withhold my kind feelings.

·

I do not have to be mean just because somebody else was. I am who I am.
I practice kindness and friendliness wholeheartedly,
because it makes me feel good
and it helps others to feel better.

·

I keep thinking of people I know. With some people,
no particular feeling arises spontaneously.
I think of them with friendliness anyway.
My goodwill and friendliness are gifts that are mine to give.

•

Breathing in, and breathing out, I now concentrate on the flow
of this positive energy through my own body.
I scan all the parts of my body, and take the time to send
loving thoughts to each part.

•

I send thoughts of kindness toward my heart, my liver,
my digestive system, and other organs.
They have worked faithfully to keep me alive and well.
I promise to be good to them in turn.
I promise to consider their health and well-being when I eat and drink.

•

There is no tension anywhere now.
With each breath, I send waves of good feelings toward
myself and others.
I relax and enjoy these good feelings.

PRACTICING WITH LOVING KINDNESS

"May all beings be happy and safe,
and may their hearts be filled with joy."

This line from the Buddha's Discourse on Loving Kindness is a meditation theme in itself. You can repeat it a few times at the beginning of your meditation period. If you can also remember to think of it during the day, it will shape your consciousness and infuse it with gentleness.

I was inspired by the Discourse on Loving Kindness when I composed the next two verses. You might enjoy including them in your evening practice:

Going to sleep tonight, I smile.
Several beautiful hours of rest are before me.
I look at all beings with eyes of compassion
And savor the last moments of this day.

And also,

Let there be peace on earth, and let it begin with me.
Let there be peace in my home, and let it begin with me.
Let there be peace in my workplace, and let it begin with me.

The world is full of self-centered people. If we hate them all, our mind would be a very disturbed place indeed. Remember that the purpose of this meditation is to bring peace by developing a loving attitude. Night is a time of peace. It is not a time for strife, anger, or settling scores, even in one's imagination. We can instead nurture a wish for all beings to be more inclusive and more loving.

I would like to end this section with a stanza in homage to the Persian poet Hafiz:

> You carry all the ingredients to turn the night into a battle—
> Don't mix them!
> You also carry all the ingredients to turn the night into a time of peace—
> Mix them, mix them!

Week Five—Time Is Now

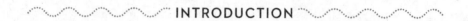

Verbs come in three tenses—past, present, and future. It is easy to extrapolate and think that there are three kinds of time corresponding to these three tenses. Indeed, when we express ourselves, we seem to talk about the past and the future as if they were time in the same sense as the present is time.

Yet there is a difference. The present moment is our home: we live in the present. We cannot live in the past or the future except in our mind, in our thoughts. Life happens in the present. Our language reflects this: a musical performance happening now is a "live" event. It is happening in "real" time.

The past and the future also exist now. They exist as memories or as expectations. They exist now in our mind. They do not exist as time in the same sense as the present is time. Once the past was time—once it was the present. Now the past is just thoughts or traces of an earlier moment. In the same way, the future is a bundle of expectations. I expect to be at work in an hour. But that is not the future—it is only an expectation. I might get stuck in traffic, a tsunami, a snowstorm, or some other impediment. The real future is not necessarily the same as the one in my thoughts.

It is essential to realize the preciousness of now. Now is the only time we are alive. Thinking takes us away from now. Our senses bring us back. The birds sing only now, and the heart beats only now. So long as we are in our senses, we are in the present. That is one of the essential differences between meditating and daydreaming: daydreams take us to another place and time away from here and now, while mindfulness meditation brings us back.

Daydreams are made of thoughts. A daydream can be like a bus. If you embark, it will take you somewhere else. There is another way of getting on the bus: the way maintenance workers get on it at the bus depot at night. They examine and observe the bus, look it over, evaluate its state, and so on. It does not take them someplace else.

Thinking has indeed become our default mode of being. I am reminded of an interview I had with one of the participants at a retreat. This person had come to discuss a roadblock he was experiencing: "I just do not seem to be able to think of the present moment," he began. "I'm always thinking of the past or the future." Indeed, as I told him, the present is to be experienced, not thought about. It is to be grasped by our senses, not by the intellect. As soon as we start thinking about it, the moment has already passed.

Thinking about the present moment had stymied another participant: "The dancer has one foot in the past [the foot she is leaping from], and one foot in the future [the foot she is landing on]. Where is the present?" Without realizing it, this participant had created a Zen koan! As long as the dancer is in her senses, she is in the present—a present that extends in both directions.

When we intellectualize about it, we can cut up the present instant into smaller and smaller slices until it disappears, and there is only the past and the future left.

Body and mind are not separate in reality. A good dancer thinks with her body. It is only when her mind separates from her body—if she starts to think about the applause she is going to get, for example—that she might get into trouble and miss her step. Body and mind are, in fact, one being. Buddha used the term *bodymind* to refer to this entity, twenty-six centuries ago. We are the ones who separate them when we start daydreaming. Mindfulness practice is there to help us heal this separation.

When we contemplate the past with mindfulness, we do not have to go to the past mentally. We stay where we are, where our body is. If we go to the past, all the feelings we once experienced will come back also. What pulls us toward the past is precisely those feelings—and some of them may be quite painful. They may also be quite sensuous or pleasant. But the past as we remember it does not exist anymore. Thomas Wolfe explores this question in his posthumously published novel *You Can't Go Home Again* (1940).

We adopt the same stance when we think about the future. Daydreaming is not the same as anticipating the future and planning for it. Here is the difference: Suppose I am about to launch a new enterprise. Daydreaming about it, I might consider how successful I will be, the expensive cars I will be able to afford, the big house I will move into, and all the good-looking people who will be happy to become my friends or sexual partners. I may even be mentally in bed with one of these beautiful people. Yet nothing is really happening. I am in an imaginary future in my mind. I am just sitting in my kitchen with the dirty dishes in the sink. The daydream is a distraction. It is a time machine. It is actually preventing me from moving on.

On the other hand, when I plan my new enterprise, I put together a convincing business plan, I make a list of local banks, make appointments to see bank managers, and so on. I stay in the present moment planning for the future. It is only by taking good care of the present that the future will be bright. The harvest will be abundant when I take good care of the garden now.

By the way, if something essential for things to go smoothly tomorrow crosses your mind while you are meditating, you might just note it down. Otherwise, your mind will keep reminding you of it, and this might get in the way of your meditation. Making a note of it is a good way to get it off your mind. Tomorrow you will not remember things that are in your short-term memory tonight.

EXERCISE

Sitting comfortably, I release my thoughts.
I let go of stress and tension and put all my attention into my breathing.

•

Breathing is all there is.
There is nothing except breathing right now.

•

There is no time apart from the breath. Breath is time.
When my attention is continuous, I experience life in its fullness.

•

Time only exists in the present. The past is not time.
Once the past was the present, but now it is only thoughts and ideas.

•

I can only live in the present.
What I think of as the future is not time. It is a bundle of expectations.

•

Past and future both exist in the present.
They exist as memories, habits, ideas, and expectations.

•

The flowers that bloomed before have left us their perfume.
That perfume exists now.

The seeds of the future are also here in the present.
Many of these seeds are underground and are invisible to me.

•

Time is embedded in my life and in my breath.
When I am one with my breath, I experience life fully
and not as an abstraction.

•

When I am one with my breath, I am always in the present.
I live in an eternal spring where all is fresh and new.

•

I am not stuck in a past made of ideas.
As I release my ideas, the past also changes for me.

•

I am grateful for being alive, I see everyone with the mind of love.
I breathe with gratitude for all the beings who support
my life and make the world beautiful.

•

Stress is not part of the future. My expectations are not part of the future.
They are part of my habits of mind.
I release these habits so that I can live with an open mind that is free.

•

Happiness is now.

There is no other time for it to be.
There is no other time.

•

I am one with my breath and with the sensations in my body.
I breathe with a peaceful heart.

Week Six—Observing the Breath

Sitting and witnessing my breath
and the song in my ears—
Witnessing that there's something tight.

Witnessing a thousand smiles,
and many more grimaces,
Witnessing big white schooners sailing in the skies.

Witnessing you walking,
and my fantasies talking,
Witnessing silent thoughts stalking.

The flowers here,
and the unspeakable cruelties there,
Witnessing my joy and my fear.

—J. E.

INTRODUCTION

Observing the breath is not the same as controlling it. This exercise starts with three deep, conscious breaths. Then, we get out of the way and let the body do the breathing. We observe only what happens.

Notice that in the last part of this exercise, we switch to observing our usual state of mind in the same vein. Like the proverbial fish in the water, we may be so used to our default mental state that we may not be aware of it. Perhaps we have always been that way, always a little anxious, a little sad or fearful. It is an important step to see our mental state objectively—it is the first step on the way to change and freedom. We cannot change something if we are not aware of it. However, we need to develop some detachment in order to be able to observe our own mind in this way. That is why this exercise comes near the end of the training.

There is a reciprocal relationship between mental states and emotions on the one hand, and thoughts on the other. Mental states give rise to certain kinds of thoughts: For example, in a lustful state, sexual thoughts keep occurring. Or, by thinking sexual thoughts, we put ourselves in a lustful state of mind.

We have more control over our thoughts than we often realize. This gives us a handle on changing our mental states. As we change our thoughts, our mental state also changes. This is also how we can cultivate a mind of love.

However, sometimes it is the other way around: a mental state changes first, and then the thoughts follow. I had a happy example of this just before I started writing these lines. I had been seeing a depressed client for coaching in mindfulness practice, and I did what I usually do with such clients: I suggested that along with MMT, she establish a regular exercise routine, and consider taking high doses of omega-3s. Unlike some others, this client took me up. She obtained her doctor's consent, consulted with a naturopath, and started a regimen of high-dose fish oil. Three weeks later, she reported that she was feeling like a new woman, and did not feel depressed anymore.

Unfortunately, high-dose fish oil does not produce dramatic results like this every time.

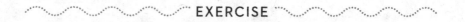

EXERCISE

I'm sitting with my back straight, my head in alignment, my legs comfortable, and my face muscles relaxed. I adjust my position as necessary so as to be comfortable.

•

*I focus on the physical sensations of breathing.
I follow the breath as it enters the nostrils and fills my lungs.
Then I exhale, and there is a pause.*

I do not control the breath or interfere.
I stay in a state of calm attention, watching the body breathing naturally.

•

When my breath is short and shallow, I notice that it is short and shallow.
When it is long and deep, I notice that it is long and deep.

•

My body does the breathing; it knows when to inhale or exhale.
I do not interfere, I just observe.

•

When I am caught up in emotions or daydreams,
my breath follows the needs of my imagination.
Now my mind is calm, and my breath is following its natural rhythm.

•

I notice that after each inhalation and exhalation, there is a brief pause.
I just wait for the breath to start again.

•

When my breath pauses at the ends,
I resist the impulse to inhale or exhale consciously.
I wait for it to happen by itself.

•

The breath has a natural rhythm like that of the waves.

Watching the rhythm of the breath is like watching
the waves on the beach.

·

There is no "I" that is doing the breathing. "I" am not responsible for it.
I remain a disinterested observer.

·

After each breath, I wait with curiosity to see when
the next breath will start again.
I wait with no expectation as to when the next breath should start.
The body starts to inhale when it is ready.

·

I enjoy this peaceful awareness of my breath.
Like the waves on the ocean, my breath has its own natural rhythm.

·

My mind is like the steady flame of a candle when
there is no wind. It is calmly aware,
not only of my breathing, but also of noises, skin sensations,
and feelings of heat or cold.

·

I note all the sensations of light and shade, of comfort and discomfort
with the same dispassionate attention.
They come and go. I only observe.

Now I observe my mental state:
Is it joyful, sad, fearful, or something else?

•

I observe the kind of mental state my mind usually serves me.
I notice whether the usual menu is worry, impatience,
regret, craving, or something else.

•

My mind has its habits.
With concentration, I become aware of my habits of mind.

Here, we are shifting away from considering our thoughts as background noise, and we start paying attention to the mind. Is fear always present? If so, can we just recognize it and not be ruled by it? Is anger often present? Why? Where does it come from? Yoga teachers sometimes talk about the "monkey mind." With this meditation, we start looking at this monkey to see what kind of an animal it is: Is it a spider monkey, a macaque, or another one of the 264 related species?

This is self-awareness—we become so used to our own mind that we take it for granted. Our quirks appear universal to us. We might even be surprised that other people do not share them. This surprise usually hits us hard when we try to live with someone.

Deep looking might have been impossible at the beginning, with the mind going every which way at breakneck speed. We cannot see the bottom of a lake on a windy day when the surface is agitated. We need to come back on a calm day. While calming the mind, we discover our sameness. We discover what a busy place the mind is. With deep looking, we discover ourselves, and we are each different in some way.

Week Seven—The Mind Is a Painter

Mind is like an artist, depicting the worlds.
If one knows that the action of mind makes
all worlds, one sees Buddha, and realizes
the true nature of Buddha.

—THE FLOWER ORNAMENT SUTRA

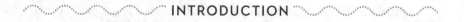

INTRODUCTION

If we get angry and all worked up about somebody while we are trying to sleep, we assume that the person who is the object of our irritation is a real person. But the real person is not in bed with us. She is somewhere else, blissfully unaware of all the commotion she is causing. What we have in bed with us is an image of that person. This image is *our* creation. We are getting all worked up about our own creation, not about a real person. If the image is a bit like a monster, it is we who have created the monster. If the image is like an angel, it is also we who have created the angel.

Like many painters, the mind emphasizes certain aspects as it creates images of people. Our feelings toward a person are based on our mental pictures, where certain features are emphasized at the expense of others. The guided meditation exercises have so far focused on taking our thoughts with a grain of salt. In this final exercise, we practice taking the image we have of a person with a grain of salt.

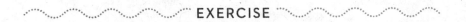

EXERCISE

*Sitting comfortably, I enjoy my breath
as my abdomen goes in and out rhythmically.*

·

*As I breathe peacefully,
my mind makes pictures of people and places I know.*

·

*I stay with my breath.
I know that these pictures are my creation.*

The people in my thoughts are fictional characters,
although they look just like the people I know.

•

I'm relaxed and I'm aware that my mind is creating a work of fiction,
a comic book, with these pictures.
I notice my mind arranging them to suit my fantasy.

•

Breathing in, I smile at these characters.
Breathing out, I know that they are not real people.
Real people have a depth that cartoon characters do not possess.

•

The fiction in my head flows on like a river.
Awareness of breath is my anchor.
It stops me from floating with the current along the river of thoughts.

•

My mind is safely tied and anchored to my body.
I am not carried along with the currents in the river.

•

I enjoy staying in my boat as it rocks pleasantly with
the waves of breath like a cradle.
I enjoy watching thoughts and images flowing by.
I remind myself that these are my own creation.

•

My mind is a good artist.
Its pictures look just like real people and places.
They are very convincing.
I breathe and smile.

•

These images are just pictures.
Any feelings I have toward them, like love, hate, anger,
or fear, are just feelings about pictures.

•

My mind deals me pictures, like cards in a card game.
Staying with my breath, I observe this game.

•

I do not choose the cards I draw.
I observe my hand and stay with my breath.

•

I am comfortable and relaxed.
I do not take this game too seriously.
I feel content.

Appendix:
Breathing from the Diaphragm

We all breathe from the diaphragm when we are sleeping, and we breathe deeply.

Despite all the hullabaloo about "the six-pack abdomen" and all the bodybuilding exercises that concentrate on the abdominals, those muscles are mostly cosmetic. The real work is done by the muscles that are in the back. That is where expressions like "backbreaking labor" come from. The back muscles keep our posture straight when we walk or sit. The muscles in the front are the breathing muscles—they work the abdomen like a bellows.

Lie on your back, put your hand on your abdomen, and cough. You will feel the abdomen contract. This is how you should breathe out. As you breathe out, the abdomen should contract, and your hand should descend. As you breathe in, your abdomen should expand, and your hand should go up.

Many people switch from one type of breathing to the other during the day. You can always check what is happening by putting your hand on the abdomen. Try this while you walk. The tummy should stay soft and go out as you breathe in. The meditating Buddha is depicted with hands crossed in the middle. This position enables the meditator to be in touch with her breathing through her forearms.

One way people tense up is by the process of sympathetic tension. This means that when you put tension on one group of muscles, other muscles join in, even though they are not involved in the action you are performing, and their contribution is unnecessary. The abdomen is considered to be an important energy center in some traditions. It is important to keep abdominal muscles from tensing up unnecessarily.

Here Is a Way You Can Train the Abdomen to Relax

- Lie on your back, and check with your hand that the abdomen is soft.
- Take a few deep breaths with your hand on your belly to establish that you are breathing from the diaphragm.
- Now try to lift one leg a few inches off the ground while you consciously prevent the abdominal muscles from contracting. The tummy should remain soft while you lift up the leg.

- If you do not succeed at first, try lifting the leg up just one inch. Then try with the other leg.
- If you have difficulty with this exercise, stop, and try again later or another day.
- The ultimate test is when you can lift both legs while the abdomen stays soft.

ACKNOWLEDGMENTS

Thich Nhat Hanh, to whom this book is dedicated, extended the Lamp of Wisdom to me and thus welcomed me into the family of Dharma teachers who are firmly rooted in the tradition. I am deeply grateful to him for his confidence and for the inspiration of his teachings. It has been a joyful and rewarding experience to share the practice of mindfulness with so many people over the years. This practice has a great deal to contribute in the fields of education, health, and ecology, and much work still remains to be done.

I appreciate Chan Huy for the enthusiasm with which he advocates the concept of Applied Mindfulness and for his Dharma friendship. Our conversations have helped me move forward at crucial times.

William Glasser, M.D., opened my eyes to a new way of looking at people and the helping relationship. My apprenticeship in his Reality Therapy counseling prepared me for seeing the interdependent nature of body and mind, of thoughts and emotions. Although I was not able to convince him of the value of the parallels between Buddhist practice and his approach to therapy in the early 1990s, I benefited hugely from his thinking.

I am indebted to Marcia Segal for revising an early draft of the book.

My literary agent, Bob Silverstein, shepherded the manuscript with loving care and much patience until it found a home with Tarcher Books. I appreciated his availability when I needed it.

Last but not least, Andrew Yackira, my editor at Tarcher, has put up with my many revisions gracefully, and has generally made the transition from manuscript to book easy. I appreciate his patience.

ABOUT THE AUTHOR

Joseph Emet lives in Montreal, Canada, and offers mindfulness mediation training sessions to individuals and groups in stress management, personal growth, and better sleep. For a complete list of current classes and workshops, please visit his website at www.mindfulnessmeditationcentre.org.

If you enjoyed this book, visit

www.tarcherbooks.com

and sign up for Tarcher's e-newsletter to receive
special offers, giveaway promotions, and
information on hot upcoming releases.

TARCHER
PENGUIN

Great Lives Begin with Great Ideas

Connect with the Tarcher Community

• • •

Stay in touch with favorite authors
Enter weekly contests
Read exclusive excerpts!
Voice your opinions!

Follow us

 Tarcher Books

 @TarcherBooks